Advocacy in Health Care

Kevin Teasdale
MA(Oxon), PhD, RMN, Cert Ed

**Blackwell
Science**

© 1998
Blackwell Science Ltd
Editorial Offices:
Osney Mead, Oxford OX2 0EL
25 John Street, London WC1N 2BL
23 Ainslie Place, Edinburgh EH3 6AJ
350 Main Street, Malden
  MA 02148 5018, USA
54 University Street, Carlton
  Victoria 3053, Australia
10, rue Casimir Delavigne
  75006 Paris, France

Other Editorial Offices:

Blackwell Wissenschafts-Verlag GmbH
Kurfürstendamm 57
10707 Berlin, Germany

Blackwell Science KK
MG Kodenmacho Building
7–10 Kodenmacho Nihombashi
Chuo-ku, Tokyo 104, Japan

First published 1998

Set in 10/12 pt Souvenir Light
by DP Photosetting, Aylesbury, Bucks
Printed and bound in Great Britain by
MPG Books Ltd, Bodmin, Cornwall

The Blackwell Science logo is a trade mark
of Blackwell Science Ltd, registered at the
United Kingdom Trade Marks Registry

DISTRIBUTORS

Marston Book Services Ltd
PO Box 269
Abingdon
Oxon OX14 4YN
(*Orders:*   Tel: 01235 465500
          Fax: 01235 465555)

USA
Blackwell Science, Inc.
Commerce Place
350 Main Street
Malden, MA 02148 5018
(*Orders:*   Tel: 800 759 6102
             781 388 8250
          Fax: 781 388 8255)

Canada
Login Brothers Book Company
324 Saulteaux Crescent
Winnipeg, Manitoba R3J 3T2
(*Orders:*   Tel: 204 224 4068)

Australia
Blackwell Science Pty Ltd
54 University Street
Carlton, Victoria 3053
(*Orders:*   Tel: 03 9347 0300
          Fax: 03 9347 5001)

A catalogue record for this title
is available from the British Library

ISBN 0-632-04977-4

Library of Congress
Cataloging-in-Publication Data
is available

Contents

Preface

This book is intended both as an encouragement and as a warning. The encouragement is because I believe that access to advocacy is still desperately needed in health care. Our systems and institutions continue to disempower the people they were intended to serve, whether these are called 'patients', 'clients', or 'service users' (I use all these terms interchangeably throughout this book). Carefully planned and expertly carried out, advocacy reminds helpers of why they came into health care in the first place and may even stand out among landmark achievements across a career. In contrast, a warning is necessary because too many sincere people have been left bruised and battered as a result of trying to stand up and be counted as advocates. I hope that the ideas and examples contained in these chapters will help potential advocates take some quite straightforward precautions to lessen the risks of advocacy for everyone involved.

I would like to think that this book has something of value in it for all health care professionals and for independent advocates as well. I hope that one of its strengths will be found in the series of genuine case histories of everyday advocacy which are used to illustrate the main points. However, it is also a weakness that these case histories are not truly representative. I collected them over several years through interviews and written questionnaires but, being a nurse myself, I had much easier access to nursing staff than to other professional groups or independent advocates. I believe that most of the learning points from the examples generalise perfectly well to the work of other groups, but I must apologise that too few of these are included in the case histories. Indeed I suspect that medical staff who read this book may easily find themselves infuriated by so many examples where they are cast in the role of opponents of advocacy. This has arisen partly from the nature of power in health care and partly as a feature of the unrepresentative range of the case histories. For the latter I again apologise and I would be very interested to hear from readers who are either independent advocates or members of any of the health care professions and who are willing to provide additional case material to improve the range in any future editions.

I would like to thank all the individuals who so willingly supplied the case histories and also Albion House Publications for permission to draw on some of the material on clinical supervision which first appeared under their imprint. Finally, I must mention that many of the ideas in this book sprang from a work-based advocacy course run at Rauceby Hospital and I would like to thank all the members of that group – Barbara Banks, Joan Carpenter, Liz Graves, Val Hall, Brenda Hanson, Mick Lowe, Larry Moore, Jean Oakes, Claire Pearce, John Southgate, Anne Spencer, Jean Thompson and Kate White – and in particular to remember Jean Savill, a strong advocate sadly missed.

Chapter 1
The Nature of Advocacy

Advocacy is about power. It means influencing those who have power on behalf of those who do not. The dictionary definition of an advocate is one who pleads, intercedes or speaks for another. In other words, advocacy is required when people feel vulnerable and powerless. It is sad but true that those who suffer from illness or disabilities frequently report precisely these feelings of vulnerability and powerlessness in their dealings with members of the caring professions. The professionals themselves have no difficulty in describing times when they interceded on behalf of patients or clients with managers, colleagues and others in positions of power. In addition, most independent advocacy organisations can recall times when they had to plead a client's cause in the face of opposition from members of the caring professions. So accepting the need for advocacy in health care as a regrettable reality, this book suggests ways in which all advocates, whether professionals or independents, can become more effective in representing the views of patients and clients, while at the same time reducing or eliminating the worst of the risks associated with advocacy. The main arguments are developed out of descriptions of real situations provided by a wide variety of people working in different types of hospital and community settings, beginning with an example of everyday advocacy from a district nurse:

'The patient lived with his wife in an isolated rural location ten miles from a doctor. He had prostate cancer and a few weeks previously had commenced on painkiller tablets. His wife was unable to accept her husband's ill health even though she had been told that his prognosis was poor. There was a great deal of stress in the home whenever I visited. The GP had increased the pain relief a day or two before, but the patient was on a variety of tablets and he found the extra ones difficult to take. Both husband and wife were upset that the doctor had not increased the strength of the tablets, only the number that had to be taken. They asked me if I would speak to the doctor on their behalf. I

1

went to see him and explained that the extra tablets were making the patient and his wife unhappy and asked would he please write another prescription for a higher strength (the prescription has to be hand-written). The GP replied that he had just that morning written out a prescription for the lower strength which was being processed in the dispensary at that very moment and it really was a lot of bother for such a little thing. He walked off.

I thought about it for a moment and then followed him. I kept calm and explained again that the couple were finding everything in life very difficult at the present time and so for them the extra tablets had become a really big issue. I asked him would he please accommodate them to make life a little easier. Begrudgingly he did so. I felt this issue was important to the patient. Small points like these represented a great part of the burden of the illness to him and his wife. I know I was at risk of alienating the doctor from myself in our future professional relationship. I could have left it after the doctor first said "no", but I felt this would have been ignoring the patient's needs for the sake of the doctor's convenience and for me to save face. I could have got the patient to contact the doctor himself and discuss it but I know he would have received a negative response. In fact the GP carried out the patient's wishes, the patient was happy about this and the doctor's fit of impatience went away quickly enough.'

This example raises many of the key issues surrounding advocacy in health care. Fundamental is the fact that one professional (in this case a doctor) was in a position of power. In our society, major drugs such as opiate-based painkillers cannot be purchased over the counter. The law decrees that, because of the risks of addiction or misuse, only individuals trusted by reason of a medical qualification may prescribe drugs based on opiates which can relieve the agony of chronic pain. As potential patients, we are all therefore beholden to the goodwill, breadth of knowledge and sensitivity of our doctors in this area. In other words, we are all potentially vulnerable and dependent, just like this man and his wife.

Yet to be a doctor is a humanitarian calling. One only enters the medical profession with a concern to lead a useful life helping others. The training and subsequent apprenticeship of a junior doctor is long and arduous. This combination of a long period of theoretical learning, plus supervision in gaining experience, is characteristic of all the professions involved in health care. Yet sometimes things seem to go wrong. What happened to make this doctor insensitive to the needs of the patient? Was it pressure of work, an unwillingness to admit a mistake, or a combination of unrelated events that left him feeling annoyed and reluctant to listen? And what of the patient and his wife – why were they reluctant to speak up for themselves? Perhaps again it is the legacy of vulnerability, with the knowledge that they would need the doctor again in the future and could not afford to alienate him. Their understanding of the illness and its treatment was limited. Yet even if they had been fully informed about these matters, our society does not permit them to act on this knowledge themselves. There may also have been an educational or social gulf between doctor and patient which hindered communication in subtle but telling ways. Whatever the case, it is clear that there was pressure on the husband and wife to use a go-between, an advocate. They chose another professional who had greater access to the doctor than they did and who also possessed some of the specialist pharmaceutical knowledge which they lacked.

The nurse in this case accepted the role voluntarily. She knew there were risks attached to it, particularly the risk of damaging her relationship with the doctor. The skill of the nurse in presenting the case was clearly important. There emerges an element of confrontation in advocacy, which can be sharpened or softened, depending on the circumstances. The district nurse appears to have used a classic calm and yet assertive approach, but this still led to a minor confrontation. It is also useful to ask what the nurse would have done if the doctor had continued to refuse her request. Advocacy frequently gives rise to ethical questions about the extent to which it is legitimate to act in a manipulative way as an alternative when assertiveness is blocked.

The district nurse's example gives us a brief glimpse into her life and work and that of the others involved in the situation. But how will the nurse's advocacy in this one situation affect work and relationships in the future? Will the doctor harbour a grudge and on some future occasion take a more determined stand against the nurse? Will the nurse be encouraged by her success to undertake more and more advocacy on behalf of patients? Will the patient and his wife come to rely on the nurse and be even less willing to speak up on their own behalf when others can do it for them? The complexities of everyday advocacy soon become evident.

The power imbalance

To anyone who has never experienced illness, it may be difficult to understand how autonomous adults holding positions of influence in the world are so willing to give up control of themselves when seeking the help of health care staff. Yet the power imbalance which determines the need for advocacy arises from all aspects of the experience of illness or trauma, both of which may be regarded as a loss of control over one's own body. In physical terms this may be experienced as a loss of consciousness or an interference with consciousness through pain, psychological disturbance and the influence of drugs used in treatment. It may show itself as a feeling of physical weakness, typified by the immobility and dependence on others which results from being bedridden. The willingness to place oneself in the hands of others and to trust them even to use knives to cut into one's body during an operation is particularly strong when events are traumatic and characterised by pain. A patient who had recently had her appendix removed and was making a successful recovery described a typical response to the emergency situation in which she had found herself:

> 'Well when I was being brought on the ambulance, I was a bit sort of anxious. Well I mean, when you've never been in hospital and you don't know what's going to happen, you tend to get a bit nervous . . . When they'd brought me in they took me into a cubicle on my own. A nurse came, then a doctor came. They sort of reassured me. Very kind to me really . . . they sort of talked to me. They tried to explain what they were going to do. You see I had to have monitoring of my heart, and one or two examinations. And they explained things that they were going to do to me before they did them . . . They didn't just bring this equipment and get on with what they were doing. They sort of explained what they were going to do.'

The striking thing about this account is the passive nature of the patient. She was 'brought on the ambulance' and 'had to have monitoring of my heart'. Things were being done that this adult did not fully understand but which she was willing to accept as being for the best. According to this account the woman was not asked to decide what would happen; her implicit consent was assumed and the explanations were given in order to reassure her rather than to help her to make decisions for herself. Professionals tend to take this degree of passivity for granted in many illness-related emergencies and in the view of this patient her recovery from the operation was convincing proof of how wise she had been to place her trust so completely in the hands of others.

Linked with physical dependence arising from illness are psychological changes. Balint (1964) argued from a psychoanalytical viewpoint that illness leads to a return to the psychological dependence characteristic of a scared child faced with an unknown threat. In this situation it is easy to give up one's autonomy and to invest almost a religious faith in powerful adult figures – described by Balint as the 'apostolic function' of the professional helpers. In addition to these physical and psychological changes, illness is characterised by new social roles. Parsons

(1951) argued that illness may be viewed as a form of deviance that our society tries to limit or control, transforming it into a 'sick role'. This is well summarised by Herzlich (1973):

> 'It is because flight into illness is a temptation for everyone that society has to exercise control over the sick and those around them. Society therefore creates roles to be played. The doctor's role is to channel in the patient the form of deviance represented by illness. The patient's role combines regressive aspects, permitted secondary gains such as freedom from responsibility and the right to assistance, with more positive types of behaviour; for instance he has his own obligations in that he must want to get better and cooperate with the doctor in seeking a cure.' (Herzlich 1973, p.8–9)

This obligation to cooperate during illness makes it more difficult for an individual to speak out and argue against the type of treatment or care ordered by the professional. The person seeking help is labelled a 'patient' and the English word itself carries a secondary meaning in relation to being 'patient' and uncomplainingly accepting the kindness and help of others. Anyone who does not accept this role risks the alternative label of 'unpopular patient' (Stockwell 1984). In any case, whenever trauma or illness necessitate admission to hospital, patients cease to exercise control over the environment in which they find themselves. The professionals organise 'the patient's day' according to routines which suit their work, even to the extent of restricting the time that a limited number of people from the outside world may come and visit.

Some aspects of hospital life, such as meals and accommodation arrangements, are labelled 'hotel services' to distinguish them from diagnostics and treatments. Yet the analogy with a hotel is far from perfect. In Britain the proud boast of the National Health Service is that its facilities are available free at the point of delivery to all who need them. This very freedom from paying for services has the side effect of encouraging yet greater passivity and dependence. In a consumer society the requirement to pay brings with it legally enforceable rights of choice and complaint about the quality of goods and services supplied. It is much harder to enforce these rights when payment is through general taxation or an insurance company.

The issue of trust

These arguments offer at least a partial explanation of the tendency of patients to be reluctant to criticise or complain about the health care services which they receive, leaving them vulnerable and dependent on the goodwill of the professionals. Many of the distinguishing features of professions in our society confer corresponding power on their members. Dingwall (1983) noted that professions rest their authority on having a specific and restricted function, while claiming to apply their knowledge in impersonal and objective ways without regard to the personal characteristics of their patients. They also claim an altruistic motivation for their services which strengthens their argument that they should be free to define their own work, to determine its method of delivery and technical content, and independently to regulate its proper conduct. Thus according to Dingwall the professions exemplify in an extreme form the role of trust as it occurs in modern societies which rely on an advanced division of labour. An eighty-three year old severely ill woman who was an in-patient in a surgical ward explains in an interview just how far this sense of trust can extend:

INTERVIEWER: 'How soon after you came into hospital did you know that ... you were going to be looked after all right, that your special needs (as a diabetic) were going to be met?'
PATIENT: 'It never occurred to me that they wouldn't be ... We are received in privacy by a group of little doctors and nurses, they ask all the questions they want, and they know all about you, and you're just in their hands.'
INTERVIEWER: 'Can you remember, did they give you any information that stayed in your memory ...?'
PATIENT: 'They give you no information except as you ask for, and if you don't ask you don't get it. I'm one of these people who isn't the slightest bit interested in any of these medical subjects. I wouldn't even know what to ask if I wanted to ask. All the asking has been done by my husband. He wanted to know everything. A malignant growth, he wanted to know things of that kind. I simply took it for granted.'
INTERVIEWER: 'And have the staff here, have they respected that ...?'
PATIENT: 'I don't think they realise. I think they say to themselves, "Oh she never asks questions". I think they take it for granted. I've always been like that with my doctor. When I'm ill I go to a doctor if I need one. I do everything he tells me. Have absolute confidence, put myself in his hands, and that's that.'

With a patient like this, advocacy is impossible. She has no desire for advocacy, nor in her eyes any need for it. Yet from the viewpoint of the staff, she is in many ways an ideal patient who creates no problems for the smooth running of the ward. Indeed there is a danger that staff can become accustomed to unquestioning attitudes like these, particularly with elderly patients. This makes it much more difficult for patients who really want to retain some control over decision-making to gain the information which would help them to monitor their condition. Thus a different patient who had a mastectomy felt very resentful about a lack of information about her prognosis:

'At a check-up someone looked at the scar and said, "That's healed nicely". But I still have a lump there and find it very uncomfortable when I try to get off to sleep. I asked how long the lump would last and was told, "It will go in time". I find people don't really answer your questions. You just get a short answer ... I asked, "What are the chances?" The doctor said, "The chances are we'll be having this conversation in five years' time". That reply didn't really tell me anything. It was a "maybe" sort of answer ... I found out more by a friend phoning a helpline and getting information. When I said this to my GP he did tell me more about my condition. He said at the hospital the specialists are too highly qualified and so they don't have the time to spend with you.'

Although the explanation given by the GP sounds like a caricature of modern medical practice, it reveals a common assumption about specialists which tends to restrict information and therefore choice. The argument that at least some of the professionals are highly qualified leads on to the view that one ought to place one's trust in them because it is impossible to match their expertise in this particular field of illness. If the specialists themselves believe this, then there is no reason to explain things to patients, other than to calm their nerves through bland reassurances. Pressures of time and workload have increased enormously within the health service, so the second part of the GP's statement adds to the pressure to conform by suggesting that asking for lengthy explanations will take up an unreasonable amount of the valuable time of the specialists, which could instead to be given to others in even greater need.

This traditional one-way view of trust was rejected by Thorne & Robinson (1988) on the basis of a series of interviews with sufferers from chronic illnesses. They found that patients increasingly looked for a relationship based on reciprocal trust as a necessary component of satisfying, effective health care. On first diagnosis, most patients had a naive trust in the professionals, but this changed as they became more aware of the chronic nature of their problems. They realised that the professionals did not fully understand their best interests and instead tried to impose their own beliefs about treatment and care. Those patients who adapted most successfully to chronic illness insisted on relationships based on mutual respect which they developed with those individual professionals who proved themselves willing to allow decisions to be made by the patients on the basis of shared understanding of treatment options and individual needs.

Many professionals, including medical staff, will feel angry when reading this and will argue that although paternalistic attitudes may characterise some of their colleagues, their own personal practice is quite different. With some justification they will say that for them the autonomy of the individual is paramount; they will offer help only with the informed consent of the patient; where there are genuine choices to be made, they will present those choices in terms the individual can understand. With a positive outlook this approach is perfectly feasible for committed professionals working with patients who are fully conscious, intelligent adults with the energy to ask questions at the right time. It becomes more problematic, however, when the patient is a child, or an elderly person with some degree of memory impairment, or an individual with a long history of illness-related anxiety. In these situations, the professional may be faced with a genuine ethical dilemma, where information which respects the autonomy of the individual may also damage the person's health. The role of the professional as an employee governed by rules and policies tends to place strict limits on allowing patients to control their own destiny when their autonomy is judged to be impaired. It also tends to support approaches which promote the smooth running of the clinical area. An example from the field of learning·disabilities illustrates the problem. The social worker who described this situation was working with clients from the wards of an old hospital due for closure once a series of new six-bed community bungalows had been built.

'I was called up and told that (my client) was on the transfer list. This client hadn't been approached about this at the time and he was a person who really couldn't cope with any sort of change. So I was a bit apprehensive about how to break the news to him. In the meantime some of his friends in the neighbouring ward had been told of the move and somewhere along the line he had been told by one of his friends that he had been included in this package. He was quite an able gentleman, he understood things. So all of a sudden he became very anxious, his behaviour became anti-social. He would come home from work and go straight to his bedroom and the next thing you would hear was all this shouting and crashing and things flying out of the door. So we were presented with this situation where he now knew there was something on the cards and we weren't too sure how to deal with him. We knew that if we said outright, "Yes you're moving in three months time", then we'd have three months of severe problems. He also stopped eating when he was anxious and would lose weight rapidly. If you served him food he'd throw it . . .

What we as a group of professional helpers came up with was a devious package which was to be implemented by all staff, where initially we were going to say, "No, you're not moving, you're staying here". I had a lot of reservations about this, telling lies to one of the clients. But we felt that purely for his wellbeing this was the correct approach. So the home opened, five clients went into the home and my client stayed on the ward. We then agreed that over a period of two to three months he would be introduced to the home. We felt that once he got to know the home and saw what a nice place it was, we could introduce him slowly. Then at the end of three months we'd say, "How do you feel about it? Would you like to live there?"

In actual fact it didn't work out at all like that. The first weekend he went over and saw one of his friends at the home. He came back full of beans: "Nice house, yes, not bad". I thought, "This is very promising". The following week he went to stay for the weekend. Once again he came back, we had no problems at all. So we thought he must be getting wise, it was going too well . . . So we got up to about the fourth week and he turned round and said, "Well actually I'd like to live there. They've got a spare bedroom." And I was absolutely bowled over. I'd been anticipating that we were going to have at least three months of inner turmoil with him. I mean, the strategy worked far better than we'd dared hope. We'd got the situation where this gentleman who would become anxious over any small change in his daily routine and the next thing he's moving house with very little problem at all.'

Taking the social worker's account at face value, the motivation of the professionals appears to be altruistic, arising from a genuine concern to act in the best interests of the client. Moreover, the successful outcome appears to justify their approach. However, a deeper level analysis may lead one to question their assessment of the capacity of the client to appreciate his own situation and to cope with changes in his life. The examples given of how the client tended to behave when anxious included shouting, throwing food and crockery. These were labelled 'anti-social' but they also presented a management problem for the staff, disrupting the routine of the ward. It is argued that this is typical of many other health care situations, in which to act beneficently by withholding information in the best interests of patients also results in easier management of patients and clinical areas. To the extent that altruism and professional self interest go together, they tend to weigh the balance against respect for autonomy and further weaken the ability of patients to secure the information they need for effective decision-making.

The argument so far has attempted to show the reasons why advocacy on behalf of patients is necessary in even the most altruistic of health services. Advocacy is rooted in an imbalance of power, in which there is real pressure on patients to suppress their doubts and fears and instead place unquestioning trust in specialist professional carers. This attitude affects the professionals who hold power, so that they can easily lose sight of the needs of individuals and become accustomed to taking decisions on behalf of groups of patients. Because of this, the role of advocacy as a counter-balance to professional power is particularly important in health care. It is perhaps surprising then that so many of those who take up advocacy are themselves professionals who are closely involved in treatment and care. The next chapter pursues this theme by examining in more detail some of the difficulties faced by health care professionals when they choose to act as advocates for their patients.

Summary of key points

- Advocacy means influencing those who have power on behalf of those who do not
- Patients are vulnerable when they enter the health care system because of weaknesses arising from their illnesses, together with lack of knowledge and very limited legal or consumer rights
- The power imbalance between professionals and patients means that the professionals can easily become accustomed to acting in a paternalistic way
- Under these circumstances many patients feel the need for more information or more help in presenting their concerns to the professional staff, especially the medical staff.

Chapter 2
The Risks of Advocacy

Because advocacy is about power, it has a potential for conflict which carries risks for all involved. These risks are comparatively low when the advocate is essentially trying to resolve a communication problem. The reasoning here is that if only the people in authority can become aware of precisely what the client wants, they will be happy to concede whatever is requested. In contrast, the risks are higher in situations where the people in authority fully understand the client's viewpoint but are not prepared to agree with it. This is no longer a communication issue, it is an argument over substance. If the advocate persists in speaking up in these cases, the argument may turn into open conflict. It may have wider ramifications, involving a clash between different professions, between males and females or between long-standing rivals. Where the advocate tries to bypass the person in authority, an old-fashioned power struggle may ensue. With such great potential for conflict, the risks to clients, to advocates and to those in authority are considerable. This chapter will highlight some of these risks by using case studies. The first one is relatively straightforward, involving a nurse who was asked to prepare an elderly patient for a cystoscopy (i.e. an examination of the bladder).

'When I said why I had come to prepare him he stated that although he realised he had signed the consent form, he did not know what the procedure was for and he didn't want it carried out. After careful explanation of what the procedure involved, the patient remained adamant that he did not want it. I called the ward doctor and explained the patient's views to him. He was obviously annoyed about this and said so to me. He then spoke to the patient to try to persuade him of the importance of the investigation but this made no difference, so the cystoscopy was cancelled and the gentleman was discharged.'

The nurse was acting as an advocate to the extent that she endorsed the patient's right to refuse the procedure and gave a supporting explanation to the doctor on the patient's behalf. However, essentially this was a low risk communication issue. Once the doctor understood the patient's views, the procedure could not go ahead. In general terms, patients' rights to refuse treatment are much stronger in both law and morality than their rights to demand treatment (Beauchamp & Childress 1979), so again there was little room for argument. Nevertheless, there were some risks involved. The nurse had to take the brunt of the doctor's annoyance. Potentially this may have had longer term consequences for the relationship between the two or it may have affected the nurse's willingness to undertake the advocate role in the future. Had the patient been persuaded by the doctor's arguments, the nurse would have been left in an awkward position for wasting the doctor's time. A recurring problem for advocates is the risk of clients changing their decisions and so undermining advocacy. From the patient's point of view, there was a risk of being labelled a timewaster and so receiving a slower response to future requests for help. The doctor, as the person in authority, risked a certain loss of face. He was the person who had interviewed the patient initially to gain written consent for the procedure. Now it could be construed that he had not done his job with sufficient care or attention. If called upon to explain the situation to his consultant, the easy options would be either to label the patient as a timewaster or to label the nurse as a troublemaker. Thus, even in straightforward communication situations, there are still risks to all the parties involved.

A more complex form of advocacy arises from a case described by an enrolled nurse working in an accident and emergency department.

'I was looking after a patient, an elderly gentleman who had been unwell over several weeks. I had carried out basic observations and then the on-call junior doctor went to see the patient. The doctor did a brief examination of the patient and then said he had a virus and was to go home, rest and take paracetamol to make him feel better. I was unhappy with this and so was the patient. I explained to the patient that I was going to have a word with the doctor on his behalf. The doctor was adamant that there was nothing more he could do, even when I suggested a referral to the senior medical officer (SMO), which he refused. I spoke to the patient asking if he would mind waiting a little while. He willingly agreed as he did not feel well enough to go home. Fortunately the patient's only relative was approximately two hours drive away, so he could not be taken home immediately. By that time a new casualty officer would be on duty. I spoke to the new doctor when he came on duty. He reviewed my patient and referred him to the SMO. I knew from experience that there was something wrong with the patient and he needed further investigations. If another casualty officer was not available, I am unsure of what action I would have taken. Throughout this episode I discussed what to do with the nurse in charge, who was in agreement. The gentleman was admitted and 24 hours later transferred to the regional renal unit with total renal failure. The original casualty officer did not comment when told what had happened. I consider the outcome of this advocacy successful and I would certainly not think twice about doing it again in any situation.'

Here the nurse acted as an advocate by pleading the cause of the patient, but was rebuffed. She was in a difficult position because as an enrolled nurse she had received only two years training and, despite her considerable clinical experience, would have been very vulnerable if the doctor had reported her for challenging his clinical judgement. She lessened the risk to herself by seeking the support of the nurse in charge, but was still left to decide how to pursue her advocacy on behalf of the patient. Her solution was not to go directly over the head of the casualty officer, but to work round him. In effect this was a manipulation of the situation based on deception – allowing the casualty officer to believe that the patient would be discharged home once his relative arrived to collect him, when in fact this was never the intention of the nurse.

After the patient had been admitted and his condition had worsened, the nurse was safe from being reported by the original casualty officer. He had seen his judgement challenged in oblique fashion and proved unsound. Whether he learned from the situation is not revealed, but there must have been a real risk of his acting unreasonably in response to future requests made by this nurse, or by other nurses. The nurse was strengthened in her resolve to manipulate future situations according to her judgement. This may be viewed as a thin end of the wedge risk to her moral values in that she might more readily resort to deception in the future. The vulnerability of the patient's position is clearly indicated in the example. He knew he felt unwell, but the person in authority was unwilling to accept this. If the nurse had been less resourceful, the patient was at risk of being discharged prematurely while suffering from a life threatening condition.

Group Advocacy

Moving further up the scale of risk, we come to situations involving advocacy on behalf of groups of patients rather than individuals. There is more of a political dimension to advocacy here, since it frequently involves challenging policy decisions taken by the most senior people in the employing organisation, people who are in position to use the disciplinary procedures of the organisation directly in order to resist unwelcome challenges. The following example of unsuccessful advocacy highlights the problems:

'One Christmas the managers wanted to close our ward, which is a 20 bedded adult and ten bedded children's ward. It was being closed for two weeks over the Christmas period. We were to be put on a surgical ward which also had pain relief patients and care of the dying. Our own children's ward has safety locks and handles and was designed specially for them. Our staff were not happy to move with the children, but the management would not take our fears as a good reason. I rang the Royal College of Nursing (RCN) to ask what course if any could be taken and was told we could write a letter stating our unhappiness at the situation and they told me the wording. I showed the letter to the staff but they were too scared to sign it or take it any further, so we did not do anything. We moved on to the new ward and it was appalling. We had a busy surgical list plus two bays of children, plus no security and only one side room for a playroom. The playroom had to be cleared one night in a hurry to accommodate a dying patient and then we had to get the body out past the children in the morning. After Christmas when we had moved back into our original ward I was taken into the manager's office and told off for ringing the RCN. But I held my ground and said they could not stop me consulting my professional body.'

If the nurse's account is accurate, who could dispute that advocacy was needed on behalf of children who could not speak up for themselves? Because the other nurses on the ward were unwilling to take the risk of protesting openly, the situation continued with evident risks to the physical and mental wellbeing of the children. The management climate appears to have been extremely hostile to challenge and the telling-off in the office suggests that the nurses were right to expect more vigorous action if they had sent the letter to the management. The managers themselves were at risk if anything serious had happened to one of the children as a result of their plan, although they might have tried to use the argument that, because the ward staff failed to bring potential problems to their notice, they were not responsible for matters of which they were unaware.

Whistleblowing

If one believes strongly in a particular cause and can anticipate harm to vulnerable people if something is not changed, acceptance of a negative decision from those in power leads to a cognitive dissonance. You

believe in the justice of the cause, you have followed the correct channels and used all your powers of persuasion, but the authorities still will
not listen. The next step, if you choose to continue as an advocate,
usually means going public. This is likely to be strongly discouraged by
the terms and conditions of most employment contracts, and consequently the risk of dismissal is high. There is an ethical dilemma in that
advocates who are employees of health care organisations cannot obey
the terms of their contracts and continue to act in what they see as the
best interests of their patients. 'Whistleblowing' is the term usually
applied to those forms of advocacy which involve going to the press and
making public something which an organisation would prefer to keep
private. It is an attempt to go over the head not just of one powerful
individual, but of a whole organisation. The charity Public Concern at
Work highlighted some of the definitions of whistleblowing in a review
of its activities (Public Concern at Work 1997):

(1) Bringing an activity to a sharp conclusion as if by the blast of a
     whistle
(2) Raising concerns about misconduct within an organisation or
     within an independent structure associated with it
(3) Giving information (usually to the authorities) about illegal and
     underhand practices
(4) Exposing to the press a malpractice or cover-up in a business or a
     government office
(5) Police constable summoning public help to apprehend a criminal;
     referee stopping play after a foul in football.

At one time whistleblowing was seen as unnecessary in a caring organisation such as the NHS. However, Virginia Beardshaw's (1981)
account of 'conscientious objectors at work', such as Ken Callanan and
Art Ramirez, changed all that. Callanan and Ramirez were student
nurses at a psychiatric hospital, who witnessed institutionalised abuse of
patients by staff. They reported what they had seen to the appropriate
nursing officers, but ward staff banded together and threatened an
industrial dispute unless the two students were banned from the wards.
The students were shunned at the hospital and were not supported by
either the management or the trades union. Callanan eventually
resigned, while Ramirez had to move to a different hospital to continue
his training. The nurse most closely involved with the abuse of patients
was eventually struck off the nursing register and an industrial tribunal
judged that Callanan had suffered constructive dismissal resulting from
the lack of support given to him.

This has not been an isolated case. A consultant haematologist, Dr

Helen Zeitlin, claimed that she was sacked after speaking in public about shortages of nurses and maintenance of standards at a hospital which was about to become an NHS Trust (Cresswell & Davies 1992). A biochemist, Dr Chris Chapman, was obliged to accept redundancy after going public on allegations of scientific and financial fraud involving senior medical staff at a British university (Hugill 1992). It was only after dropping an industrial tribunal case against his former employers that he was re-employed (Health Service Journal 1993). These headline cases represent a wider problem, as Hunt and Shailer (1995) found in a survey of whistleblowing in the health service. Thirty people admitted whistleblowing, of whom twenty-two were nurses or midwives, five were doctors and three were other health professionals. The categories of complaint which they reported included inadequate care, staff shortages, patient abuse, fraud or theft, poor practice, unethical research and unfair treatment of members of staff.

The majority of them began by speaking or writing to their managers. They tended to start the process in the belief that the problem was one of communication rather than substance and mainly undertook their actions as individuals, rather than in a group.

'The quantity and nature of the evidence obtained by the employee to support the case being made was very variable. In some cases, believing that management (usually at a low level) would readily believe what the complainant had to say, the complainant made little effort to gather evidence in any form. Faced with unexpected rebuttals the complainants then found themselves at a disadvantage in making the case. Going back to gather evidence, they then found that it had been "concealed".' (Hunt & Shailer 1995, p.7)

Almost one third of the group reported various forms of intimidation, including warnings about career prospects and future employment; one quarter reported that the major obstacle was simply passivity or disbelief; three said their suspension prevented them from pursuing their concern; a further three said that they received threats of violence from colleagues implicated in allegations; four said they were put under surveillance by management; three more were labelled sick or unable to cope; and two complained that managers and senior colleagues deliberately closed ranks against them.

The risks to these advocates included 23 counter-complaints against them. Most commonly these were about unprofessional conduct, including being uncooperative, not complying with management instructions and breaching confidentiality. Two were accused of having damaged the reputation of their institution, three were accused of abusing or neglecting patients and three were questioned about their sexual conduct or preferences. Of the 30 people who responded to Hunt & Shailer's survey, 17 had gone public, mostly by contacting the media. More than half the group had either lost their jobs or felt obliged to resign as a consequence of their whistleblowing.

The case of Graham Pink

Probably the best known case of whistleblowing in the NHS in recent years is that of Graham Pink (Mihill 1991). Mr Pink was a night duty charge nurse working on a geriatric ward for acutely ill patients. He became concerned at the lack of staff and poor working conditions on the ward and determined to plead the cause of the patients who were unable to speak out for themselves. He used the formal channels of the hospital to bring the situation to the notice of senior managers but with no effect. He then stepped up his campaign by writing to the local health authority and to his MP. In one letter he wrote:

'Two weeks ago, one of our staff nurses had a quite harrowing and arduous night during which three patients died in as many hours. Such was the pressure on the staff that we could not prevent one group of relatives, whose mother was still breathing, from having to move aside while the mortuary trolley was brought past them.'

In another letter he stated that,

'A very feeble and ill lady (was) being pushed into the day room on admission and left there for an hour because a corpse was in the bed she was to occupy, while I had to lie to the relatives. It amounts to a catalogue of shame and neglect which must be brought into the open for our whole community to know of, if need be.' (Chaudhary 1991)

Despite these letters and the explicit threat of going public, Graham Pink remained dissatisfied with the response from the management. He contacted *The Guardian* newspaper which published the series of letters that he had written. Following further contacts with a local newspaper, he was suspended under allegations that he had broken patient confidentiality, failed to attend a disciplinary hearing and failed to report an accident involving a patient (Mihill 1991). The charge of breach of confidentiality arose from a complaint by relatives about an interview which he gave to a local newspaper. The relatives said that although the names of patients were changed in the article, it was possible to identify their loved one from the details of care given. Graham Pink was called before a disciplinary committee of the health authority and a final written warning was issued. He was also informed that he was to be transferred to a new post in the community, which to Graham Pink appeared tantamount to constructive dismissal. In addition, he was reported to the professional conduct committee of the UKCC, the governing body of the nursing profession. Interestingly, although he had lost the disciplinary hearing run by the health authority, the professional conduct committee found that he had no case to answer and fully supported his continued registration as a nurse.

The pattern of risk in Graham Pink's case follows that described by Hunt & Shailer (1995). He at first believed that the problem was one of communication and once the management had seen conditions for themselves they would surely act. He soon discovered resistance to the substance of his complaints and was then placed in a disturbing ethical dilemma over loyalty to his patients and his profession against loyalty to his employers. By going public to a national newspaper, he placed his own job at risk. He soon faced counter-charges which left him vulnerable to a disciplinary hearing in which his employers acted as both judge and jury. The risk of breaching confidentiality and distressing others was a real one. The relatives who complained about the local newspaper account were angry and hurt as a result of the article. The hospital itself and the senior managers employed there also had their reputations damaged by the sequence of events.

Whistleblowing and the law

The legal position for staff who take their advocacy as far as Graham Pink is not particularly supportive. All employees who have been in post for a specified minimum period have a right not to be unfairly dismissed under employment protection legislation (Thorold 1981). This means that an employer could be challenged in an industrial tribunal to show that there was a legally sound reason for the dismissal and that the disciplinary process was conducted fairly. The law extends only to limited financial compensation if an employer's actions are found to have been unfair. However, by going public about a complaint, an employee may be deemed to have breached the trust or confidence which could reasonably have been expected from him.

'Under employment law the values to which importance is attached – loyalty, obedience, confidentiality and deference – inevitably conflict with the interests of the press, and the frontiers of the law are far more influenced by the former than the latter. An employee who is disciplined ... should anticipate that if what he does brings public disrespect or suspicion on his employer or the institution in which he works, the onus may be on him to justify the apparent violation of the legally proper norms of behaviour.' (Thorold 1981, p.77)

Many professions have codes of conduct which place a duty on their members to protect the interests of patients and to act as advocates on their behalf when they are unable to do so for themselves. These codes may serve to protect the professional registration of whistle-blowers such as Graham Pink, but they have no direct force in employment law. This means that advocates may retain the support of their professions while suffering the loss of their jobs. The risks to advocates increased in Britain in the late 1980s and early 1990s when NHS Trusts began to take on some of the characteristics of the world of business by competing in the internal market of the health service (Teasdale 1992a). Trusts which lost the confidence of the public or which had their reputations damaged in the press found it more difficult to maintain their contracts with the GP fundholders and health authorities which controlled their income. In this climate, employers began to tighten the terms of the employment contracts to include gagging clauses forbidding contact with the press. A draft NHS code of confidentiality issued in 1994 met a storm of protest over claims that it lacked substance and would not bolster even the existing inadequate safeguards (Cross 1994).

Reviewing the situation as a whole, it seems surprising that any health care employee should take on an advocacy role when the risks are so great and the support available so weak. Yet the detailed examples of advocacy which have been cited serve to illustrate the powerful emotional identification with patients which can lead professionals to ignore the risks. It is their closeness to human suffering which helps to explain why some professionals will always feel impelled to weigh the needs of patients above duty to their employers and so pursue a course of advocacy whatever the risks.

Summary of key points

- Advocates deal with both communication problems and issues of substance
- Serious conflict tends to arise when people in authority are reluctant to accept the substance of the patient's case
- Advocacy on behalf of a group of patients is particularly likely to turn into an argument over issues of substance

- Strong emotional identification with patients can lead advocates to blow the whistle and go public
- Whistleblowing is particularly risky for professionals, who are vulnerable to dismissal and who have very limited protection under employment law.

Chapter 3
Types of Advocacy

The discussion so far has centred on advocacy by professionals on behalf of patients. However, this is not the only type of advocacy. Among the different types listed by Gates (1994) are self-advocacy, citizen advocacy and collective advocacy. This chapter begins by outlining each of these three types and then goes on to explore the comparison with advocacy by health care professionals.

Self-advocacy

> 'In self-advocacy people are encouraged to speak up for themselves, thus bringing about an element of self-empowerment, that is, people speaking for themselves rather than having an advocate speak for them.' (Gates 1994, p.4)

Self-advocacy has drawn particular attention in the field of learning disabilities where it has helped to shift attention away from doing things for individuals and towards helping them to present their own concerns. Most typically self-advocacy involves setting up groups where members can identify common problems and support one another in deciding how to put forward their views. Very often there are non-disabled members in the group as well, who may be health care professionals with a commitment to empowering their clients. In mental health the pattern is similar, with an emphasis on user-groups within discrete services, such as day care units, where the groups are encouraged to state their views on the way the organisation is run and which act as a body for consultation when major changes are proposed by the service providers.

However, there is no reason why self-advocacy should be limited only to learning disabilities and mental health. The idea applies equally to any attempt to support and empower patients to speak up for themselves. Individual patients in general hospitals engage in self-advocacy when they assertively request additional information before making decisions

21

about treatment options. Dawson and Palmer (1991) state that self-advocacy is about speaking out and speaking up, taking responsibility for yourself, knowing what the choices are and being able to choose, disagreeing with people without being thought of as a troublemaker and being confident and assertive. These ideas are relevant to all who are made vulnerable by reason of illness as well as disabilities.

Citizen advocacy

Citizen advocacy originated in the USA, emerging from their strong libertarian tradition with its emphasis on the rights of the individual. In the UK it is more frequently termed independent advocacy. Gates (1994) describes an early example arising from a conference on cerebral palsy in 1966 when a number of ageing parents expressed worries about the continuing welfare of their children after their deaths. It was suggested that a citizen advocacy service should be established to represent the children in their future dealings with health care organisations and other services. A condition of becoming citizen advocates was that individuals should be unpaid and unconnected with the care services provided for the children. The aim was to make the advocates as independent as possible in their role of speaking out on behalf of individual children.

An extension of this idea was made by Wolfensberger (1972) who said that citizen advocates deal with two types of need, instrumental and expressive. Instrumental needs are things required for the practicalities of everyday living, for example financial support, access to appropriate health care services and living environments adapted to meet personal requirements. Expressive needs are about friendship, security, love and belonging. For Wolfensberger therefore citizen advocacy meant establishing a long term partnership with an individual, operating at an emotional level as well as a practical level.

These themes have persisted in the independent advocacy movement in the UK, although most developments still arise in the fields of learning disabilities and mental health. In general health care, advocates or patients' representatives have been established in general practices and in the nursing or administration areas of some general hospitals. The level of independence of these posts varies and in some cases existing members of staff are employed in a new capacity in order to represent patients in dealing with complaints (Mallik 1997).

Collective advocacy

Collective advocacy is sometimes called 'class advocacy' and refers to an organised group of people campaigning for a particular cause.

MENCAP, MIND and Help the Aged are major UK charities working for specific groups of vulnerable people and aiming to improve the quality of their lives through publicity and campaigning action. These organisations will offer advocacy for individuals at times, following citizen advocacy models, but their major remit is at a political or policy development level. A charity which offers both types of advocacy is Public Concern at Work. They give a free and confidential advice service to individuals who have concerns about serious wrongdoing which threatens the public interest. They function as a legal advice centre, which means that individuals can talk to them without technically breaching their employment contracts or duty of confidence to their employer. Their particular campaigning stance is to try to make it safer and easier for people to bring serious concerns to the attention of employing organisations, arguing that whistleblowing is essential to the accountability and long-term success of business (Public Concern at Work 1997).

Pros and cons of different types of advocacy

The most extensive literature on health care advocacy arises from a debate within the largest profession, nursing, about the pros and cons of professional advocacy as opposed to independent advocacy or self-advocacy. The debate is worth summarising since its main themes apply to advocacy by an employee of any health care profession and not just to nurses. The principal arguments in favour of advocacy by professionals centre on the professionals' availability, their relationship with service users and their technical and personal knowledge of the health care systems. Members of all the health care professions, including medical staff, regularly speak out on behalf of vulnerable patients. Most of this is one-off or issue-specific advocacy, representing patients' views to colleagues, other professionals or agencies outside the health service. The professionals claim close day to day contact with individuals or, in the case of GPs, a relationship with a family which may extend over many years. The professionals argue that their technical knowledge of health, illness and the range of treatment options places them in a good position to give detailed information to vulnerable people and to help them to appreciate the full range of choice which is open to them. They also argue that they understand the health care system that employs them and therefore they know how best to approach different departments or specific colleagues in order to plead a cause.

Table 3.1 shows arguments for and against advocacy. The counter arguments to advocacy by professionals claim that professionals lack objectivity and are hamstrung by being paid by the employing

Table 3.1   Advocacy in nursing – for and against.

For advocacy	Against advocacy
Part of daily activities of the nurse: Albarran (1992) and Segesten (1993)	Much of what nurses claim as advocacy is non-mandated and paternalistic; patients may be used as pawns in professional power games: Allmark & Klarzynski (1992)
A professional role of the nurse: Cabell (1992), Carpenter (1992), Clarke (1989) and Jenny (1979)	Nurses lack power within the system: McFadyen (1989) and Kendrick (1994)
Part of the human and therapeutic relationship between nurses and patients: Copp (1986) and Morse (1991)	Nurses are too much part of the system to have the independence required of an advocate: Melia (1989) and Porter (1988)
Nurses know the system: Fay (1978) and Graham (1992)	Advocacy properly defined involves a longer-term relationship than most nurses can give: Wynne-Harley *et al.*
Nurses well placed to act as mediators: Jones (1982) and Nelson (1988)	
Nurses have a commitment to act when patients ask for their help: Teasdale (1994)	
Nurses and patients both lack power and so are natural allies: Winslow (1984)	

In the middle

There is a role for advocacy within the limited power which nurses possess: Becker (1986)

Nurses can only be effective as advocates if they have personal qualities such as an ability to tolerate uncertainty and determination: Brower (1982)

Nurses can only act as advocates if they have sufficient knowledge and skills, including assertiveness, knowledge of ethics and of the law: Cahill (1994), Morrison (1991), Robinson (1985), Sutor (1993) and Webb (1987)

Arguments against are that patients are too dependent on nurses for a truly voluntary mandate; nurses lack the knowledge and skills; nurses are not independent enough. Argument for is that patients have human rights and nurses have a duty to uphold these: Castledine (1981)

Nurses tend to adopt an advocacy role too readily without considering the value for patients of independent advocacy: Gates (1995)

Advocacy, especially whistleblowing, is particularly risky for nurses and they should consider using agencies outside their employing organisation: Mallik & McHale (1995)

Nursing advocacy can only be effective when power is delegated by the institution or by medical staff or consumers: Miller *et al.* (1983)

organisation which has an interest in the status quo (Wynne-Harley *et al*. 1996). These counter arguments also support the claims of independent advocacy or self-advocacy. It is proposed that professionals lack the time for longer-term relationships with vulnerable people. Certainly in the medical and surgical wards of general hospitals, the average length of stay is far shorter than formerly and for many patients it is no more than a few days, with day surgery reducing contact time with the professionals to a matter of hours. However, in mental health and learning disabilities, contacts tend to last much longer and with community care may in some cases extend over years. A slightly different line of counter-argument is that the professionals care for many people at a time and so individual patients may be reluctant to permit a close relationship to develop when the professionals' attention is necessarily shared between so many.

The conflict of interest which professionals may experience between their duty to patients and their duty to their employer has already been highlighted. From the patients' point of view, professional staff may not be seen as potential advocates because they are regarded as part of the system. Some writers have also argued that non-medical groups such as nurses are themselves disempowered by a medically governed health care system (McFadyen 1989; Miller *et al*. 1983). They claim that if professionals lack decision-making power, they may be unable to take appropriate action on behalf of patients when reasoned persuasion fails. Castledine (1981) cited three additional arguments against non-medical professionals (specifically nurses) as advocates:

> 'First, the nurse's unique role results in the patient being forced to be dependent on her for fear of pain and suffering. Second, the general educational background of most nurses is inadequate ... Third, the patient has little choice of who is to act as his advocate.'

Finally, it is claimed that the relationship between the professional and the patient cannot be one of equality, when so much of the information and organisational knowledge is retained by the professional.

My view is that all these arguments have some relevance and need to be taken into account in advocacy situations, but that the sheer volume of contacts which professionals have with patients and the vulnerability of so many people once they enter a health care system means that caring professionals will be drawn into advocacy whether they like it or not. However, this is not a universally accepted viewpoint, even within the professions themselves (Wynne-Harley *et al*. 1996). Part of the problem relates to how advocacy is defined and in many of the debates it turns out that different parties are using the word 'advocacy' to mean very different things.

Definitions of advocacy

A useful starting point is Maggie Mallik's (1995) analysis of the health care literature on advocacy, particularly the nursing literature. Using bibliometric methods, Mallik analysed the size and growth of writing about advocacy from 1976 onwards. She linked the history of health care advocacy with the American concern for patients' rights which arose in the aftermath of the civil rights movement of the 1960s.

'American nurses saw themselves as taking on a new role and were keen to portray themselves as the patient's advocate. The UK material cited was an eclectic mixture that did not follow any set pattern but focused on some areas of concern over patients' rights without actually ever using the word "rights" until 1980 and then only twice.' (Mallik 1995, p.13)

The late 1970s and early 1980s saw some American thinkers writing influential accounts of the nature of advocacy (Curtin 1979; Gadow 1980a; Kohnke 1982). These stimulated increased interest in the topic and between 1981 and 1986 advocacy citations averaged 175 per year, with a widening emphasis on patients' rights and the consumer movement on both sides of the Atlantic.

This interest has been maintained in the 1990s, although the UK literature has begun to diverge from the North American in its view of what advocacy means. The North American view is most clearly expressed by Kohnke (1982) who takes the dictionary definition of defending or pleading the case of another but says that this describes the situation which exists when patients are very young or unconscious or for some other reason unable to act on their own behalf. She says that this definition does not apply to advocacy in general, nor to most of the situations which nurses encounter in their professional practice where most patients are conscious and can speak up for themselves. Kohnke explains her position:

'Briefly, the role of the advocate is to inform the client and then to support him in whatever decision he makes. This type of support differs from the support provided by a lawyer. In the practice of law, the lawyer advocate actually presents the client's case and either pleads for justice or defends the client from accusation. In the nurse advocate role, however, support means that when the client makes a decision, the nurse abides by it and defends his right to make it. The role of advocate comprises only two functions: to inform and to support.' (Kohnke 1982, p.2)

This definition is essentially self-advocacy. According to Kohnke the role of the professional is to provide the amount and type of information which patients want and then to support them in making their decisions, for example about treatment options. She is quite clear that even the supporting role does *not* extend to fighting patients' battles for them. For the professionals it is limited to reassuring patients that they do not have to give in to pressure from others to change their decisions, and not applying such pressure themselves where they disagree with the patient's choice: 'Approving of patients' decisions is not required by the advocate role; you are required only to accept their right to make them' (Kohnke 1982, p.28). 'Rescuing' is the term that Kohnke reserves for going out and pleading a case on behalf of patients instead of allowing them to perform this function for themselves. Kohnke's justification for this limited definition of the advocacy role of the professional is twofold. In part it springs from a belief in the importance of individual autonomy based on the claim that it is better for people to take responsibility for themselves than for someone else to take over in a beneficent way; the second justification for limiting advocacy is Kohnke's analysis of the risks of speaking out and her view that it is far less risky for patients than for nurses to do this, because patients have clear rights whereas staff are vulnerable to counter-charges from other professionals and managers.

An illustration of these points comes from the case of a registered nurse, Jolene Tuma, working in Idaho in the United States (Kohnke 1982, p.23–24, p.116). Tuma was caring for an elderly woman suffering from leukaemia. The consultant explained the need for chemotherapy and its side effects. The patient agreed to take these drugs but later told Tuma that she had doubts about them. Tuma explained a range of alternative forms of treatment and the patient indicated a preference for one of them. However, she asked Tuma to explain them also to her son to help her to make her choice. Tuma did this, but without informing the consultant of what she was doing. The son told the consultant who brought charges against Tuma, accusing her of interfering in his professional relationship with his patient. Tuma was found guilty of 'unprofessional conduct' and suspended by the state board of nursing. This decision was later overturned on technical grounds. Kohnke cites the case as an example of the risks a nurse can face in information giving. However, she criticises Tuma on two points. First Tuma should have told the consultant what she was doing so that he could have had an opportunity to explain matters himself. Second,

Tuma was engaging in 'rescuing' by agreeing to talk to the son. She should have encouraged the patient to speak to the son herself and supported her in undertaking this.

Kohnke's view that advocacy should be limited to merely informing and supporting patients is challenged by British writers such as Maggie Mallik (1995). She argues that the most usual form of advocacy is 'triadic', meaning that it involves three parties, the patient, the advocate and another person whom patient and advocate wish to influence. Mallik conducted focus group interviews with practising nurses who had no difficulty in recalling examples of what they called advocacy when they attempted to influence a third party on behalf of patients. They did not regard this as 'rescuing' but as a necessary human aspect of caring and they recognised that there was an element of conflict built into these situations. Some of their patients were what Curtin (1979) termed 'silent' in the sense that they had difficulty speaking up for themselves. Mallik found that the silent category went beyond children and unconscious people mentioned by Kohnke (1982) and extended to many elderly people as well as younger adults whose limited energy, education or self confidence made it impossible for them to speak out. In fact Mallik found very few examples of self-advocacy or empowerment where the nurse's role was limited to information or support; most of her nurses described pleading or defending a cause.

The problem of silent patients

The problem of silent patients needs to be addressed in more detail. To understand the issue fully it is important to have a grasp of some of the principles of medical ethics which may influence decision-making in health care. Beauchamp & Childress (1979) provide an overview of these principles, picking out four which they claim are accepted by all mainstream theories of ethics as guides to ethical decision-making:

- Justice
- Respect for autonomy
- Beneficence
- Non-maleficence

Justice means treating equals equally. So in terms of advocacy it strongly supports non-discriminatory approaches under the principle that a person's race, gender, creed, etc. are not relevant in decision-making about the health needs of the individual. Justice is also the principle supporting the claims of most collective advocacy action groups.

The second principle, respect for autonomy, means that:

'insofar as an autonomous agent's actions do not infringe the autonomous actions of others, that person should be free to perform whatever action he wishes – even if it involves serious risk for the agent and even if others consider it to be foolish.' (Beauchamp & Childress 1979, p.59)

In relation to advocacy, this principle supports the patient's right to information about treatment or care that will permit informed choices to be made. It also adds weight to Kohnke's (1982) argument that advocates should support the decisions made by their patients, regardless of whether or not they agree with them.

In contrast, the principle of beneficence is the duty to do good to other people, while non-maleficence is the duty to do no harm to others. One of the main problems with beneficence and non-maleficence is that they can easily lead to paternalistic actions in which the professionals present information and make decisions in what is seen as the best interests of the patients, thus relegating them to the status of children under benevolent parental authority. My interpretation of Kohnke is that, even in cases where professionals believe that patients' decisions will cause them harm or deny them benefit, she argues that respect for autonomy should take priority over any ideas of further intervention in the name of beneficence or non-maleficence. This contrasts with the legal position on consent to treatment in England and Wales that was established by the Sidaway case, where the appeal court allowed doctors to withhold information if in their clinical judgement it would be detrimental to patients to disclose it (Elliott Pennels 1998). This denies patients (and those who advocate on their behalf) any legal right to informed consent, leaving the judgement of what to disclose as that which a reasonable body of professionals in the same specialty would tell patients.

Further difficulties for advocates occur when individuals are not autonomous. One of Mallik's (1995) focus group nurses recounted a situation in theatre when a patient was already anaesthetised. The nurse halted the procedure and insisted that the patient was moved into a safer position. The doctor involved threatened to report her for interfering but she insisted on grounds of health and safety and he backed down, although he continued to harass her afterwards. The nurse could say that she was trying to prevent harm to the patient and so obeying a duty of non-maleficence. But was this advocacy? She could argue the case in the sense that she was publicly defending the patient against harm, yet there was no opportunity for prior information-giving or patient choice in the matter and there was no sense in which the patient had explicitly delegated an advocacy role to the nurse. The nurse involved certainly regarded this as advocacy. Certainly there was nothing paternalistic about her actions, which aimed to defend the patient's right to avoid harm and presumably the patient would have supported the nurse's intervention if conscious when it occurred. So if we accept this as a valid example of advocacy, then it follows that when dealing with 'silent' patients the usual requirement to give information and support decision-making does not necessarily apply, nor in this situation was it necessary for the patient explicitly to request advocacy from the professional.

Clearly there are risks here of professionals taking it on themselves to define the advocacy needs of silent patients in terms of their own prejudices and beliefs, or to use advocacy for patients as an excuse for fighting personal feuds. A nursing advisory document picks out these concerns in a section on advocacy (UKCC 1989). It defines advocacy as concerned with promoting and safeguarding the wellbeing and interests of patients and clients. It states that advocacy involves professionals in helping patients by making such representations on their behalf as they would make themselves if they were able. The booklet goes on to explain advocacy as a positive and constructive activity which is integral to good professional practice, but not one which is concerned with conflict for its own sake. The guidelines allow for professional judgement in deciding when and how advocacy should be exercised, insisting that 'the practitioner must be sure that it is the interests of the patient or client that are being promoted rather than the patient or client being used as a vehicle for the promotion of personal or sectional professional interests' (UKCC 1989, p.12). Arising from these guidelines is the issue of how to assess the interests of patients, together with a whole range of questions about decision-making in advocacy which are the subject of the next chapter.

Summary of key points

- Advocacy may be classified into four types:
  (1) Self-advocacy
  (2) Independent or citizen advocacy
  (3) Collective, class or group advocacy
  (4) Advocacy by professionals.

- Each type has its own strengths and weaknesses
- Writers from the USA tend to argue that the only valid type of advocacy is self-advocacy
- Most of the literature from the UK supports a broader definition of advocacy which embraces all four types.

Chapter 4
An Advocacy Flowchart

In Britain and North America, advocacy is closely associated with the concept of patients' rights. Particularly important among these rights are those supported by the ethical principle of respect for autonomy, namely the right to information and the opportunity to exercise choice over treatment or care. In ethical terms, one person's right is another person's duty. So to the extent that a right to information or choice of treatment is conceded by the professionals, they then have a duty to supply information and explain choices. However, many users of health care services are likely to have difficulty exercising their rights without help, because their illness or disabilities effectively reduce their autonomy, at least in the eyes of the professionals. Also both the prestige and the authority of professional staff, particularly on their own territory in hospitals or clinics, make it even harder for vulnerable individuals to access information or make meaningful choices.

Controversies

Advocates try to help patients to voice their concerns. The advocates may be the patients themselves using self-advocacy, or they may be relatives or friends, health care professionals or independent advocates. In recent years much of the debate on advocacy in health care has become polarised into arguments about which type of advocacy is the best. This is essentially a sterile controversy in which the only answer is, 'It all depends on the circumstances'. There are times when the knowledge and influence of professionals make them the most effective advocates; there are times when the independence and objectivity of citizen advocates are essential; and there are times when patients do better to represent themselves, or to get their relatives or friends to act for them. What we need is a deeper understanding of the circumstances which favour each approach, rather than a simplistic search for a single best solution.

The second area of controversy is the argument mentioned in

Chapter 3 between North American and British authors over the limits of advocacy. The North American view is that a narrow definition of advocacy should be adopted, limiting activity to giving patients information and then supporting them in making their own decisions. The reasons quoted in support of this advice are that it is better for patients to be empowered and learn to act for themselves, an approach that is also less risky for the professionals. In contrast, the British authors propose a broader definition of advocacy which can encompass information giving and supporting patients, but which also extends to pleading or defending their cause in the presence of third parties. The reasoning behind this approach is that it is consistent with the everyday use of the word 'advocacy', it addresses the issue of how to promote the rights of silent patients, and there is plenty of evidence that this is what professionals actually do in practice.

On analysis, this debate over the limits of advocacy is about exactly the same thing as the argument over the different types. The North American authors are proposing that self-advocacy is best in all circumstances, so the helping agencies should concentrate on empowering patients and clients. In contrast, the British writers are saying that external advocates (whether relatives and friends, professionals or independent advocates) are also necessary. The view proposed in this book supports a broad interpretation of advocacy in the sense that I believe all the different types have something to offer to people in need. The learning point from the controversies is that it is better to move on and see advocacy as a multi-agency activity. We need to support all the different types and to try to make them mutually compatible so that they offer real choice for patients.

The flowchart

To take this a stage further, the flowchart in Fig. 4.1 specifies the decisions which face a helper who is trying to decide whether or not advocacy is appropriate for an individual client. The flowchart is based on analysis of over 150 critical incidents reported by a variety of health care professionals from their clinical practice. The first question posed is whether the client is capable of making a choice about wants. The term 'wants' is deliberately used in preference to 'needs' because 'needs' tend to be ascribed to clients by helpers, whereas 'wants' are expressions of the feelings of the individual clients themselves. The starting point for advocacy is therefore rooted in the way clients see their situation, and their own judgements about what will help them. It is supported by the ethical principle of respect for autonomy.

Figure 4.1 poses a simple yes/no answer to the question about

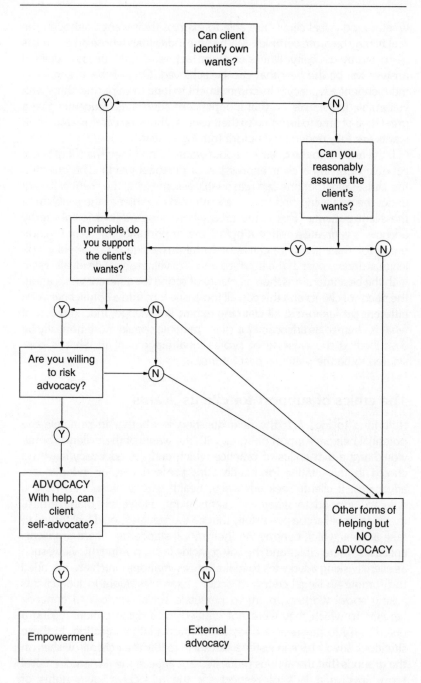

Fig. 4.1 An advocacy flowchart.

whether individual clients are able to express their wants, although the reality may be more complex. With some individuals whose autonomy is restricted by disability, illness or other factors, a cautious and qualified answer will be the best that can be achieved. One of the strengths of independent advocacy is its commitment to long term partnerships with vulnerable individuals, so that independent advocates frequently give a great deal of time to listening to their clients, checking carefully that their wants are fully understood before moving forward.

If the answer to the question about wants is 'no', then the client is not capable of giving a clear expression of personal wants. The question then arises whether one can reasonably assume what the client will want under the prevailing circumstances, referred to earlier as the problem of the silent patients. This is the area where the potential for abuse by advocates is greatest, since it opens the opportunity for them to campaign for their favourite cause or to take revenge on unpopular colleagues under cover of the ascribed needs of vulnerable individuals. Even with the best intentions there is plenty of scope for different views about the needs of clients and this can all too easily turn into a conflict between different professionals, all claiming expert knowledge. Indeed much of what is claimed as advocacy for silent patients should more honestly be described as the exercise of professional judgement in what is considered to be the patients' best interests.

The ethics of support for clients' wants

Returning to Fig. 4.1, the next question is whether in principle the potential helpers support or agree with the wants of their clients. Some would argue that codes of practice which endorse advocacy leave no choice in this matter for health care professionals or independent advocates; if clients seek advocacy, health care professionals have a duty to respond to whatever clients want. However, many ethical theorists would argue powerfully that no individuals should feel forced to take actions which contravene their moral standards. There are clear-cut cases where ethics and the law coincide in supporting this view, such as clients asking advocates to make representations which are intended to promote an illegal course of action. Examples might include clients asking social workers to try to persuade social services to concede benefits to which they were not entitled; or a dying patient asking a nurse to try to persuade a doctor to deliver a lethal injection. In these situations advocates can justify a refusal to follow their clients' wishes on the grounds that the actions requested are against the law and in moral terms involve a lack of respect for the advocates' own rights of autonomy.

However, in practice advocates are more likely to be faced with borderline situations where the legal position is not an issue. An example given by a palliative care nurse helps to highlight the problem:

'The patient was a woman with bowel cancer who had been maintained well for five years when her lungs became involved, leading to breathlessness and fear. She came into hospital but then asked me to persuade the doctors to let her go home. I told her that I thought it would not be a good idea for her to go home right now and that I didn't agree with speaking to the doctors. I asked her to remember how frightened she was when she was last at home and breathless. I told her that the doctors wanted to stabilise her and she seemed to accept this. I only gave the woman a partial explanation of why she should stay in hospital, because I didn't want to hurt her with bad news about her chances. I discussed this situation with a colleague who supported my approach. I probably could have persuaded the doctors to discharge her, but in my professional judgement the woman would have died a very frightening death, suffocating at home. As it happened, she weakened rapidly and died peacefully.'

The patient asked the nurse to act as an advocate on her behalf and the nurse refused. The question is whether she was morally or professionally justified in refusing. The argument against her refusal is that she was making a judgement about what was right for the woman without fully consulting her or explaining the position to her. The nurse admitted that she withheld some information. To this extent the nurse was not fully respecting the woman's autonomy. A second argument against her refusal is that the nurse was going against the guidelines on exercising accountability issued by her professional body (UKCC 1989). However, the guidelines can be interpreted in different ways. On the one hand they state that the exercise of professional accountability involves making representations on behalf of patients that the patients would make for themselves if they were able. But the guidelines also state that nurses must decide for themselves precisely how advocacy is to be satisfied within their own spheres of practice. In addition, the guidelines are set firmly within the context of a code of conduct which begins with a duty to safeguard and promote the interests of individual patients and clients (UKCC 1992).

This can be used to support one of the moral defences of the nurse's actions: that she was acting in what she considered to be the best interests of the patient by turning down her request for advocacy. In ethical terms the nurse believed that the principle of non-maleficence, or not doing harm, carried greater weight than the principle of respect for autonomy in this particular situation. Her clinical knowledge led her to judge that:

(1)   The woman was close to death
(2)   The level of support that could be provided at home would be insufficient to prevent the appearance of frightening symptoms
(3)   A peaceful death could be achieved if the woman stayed in hospital.

Thus the nurse appeared to believe that her actions were justified as safeguarding the woman from a frightening death.

One could argue that the nurse should have explained the situation more fully to the patient to allow her to make up her own mind. The nurse said she decided against this because she did not want to alarm the patient further. This is certainly not treating the patient as a fully autonomous individual, but more information about the physical and emotional state of the patient would be needed to allow us to judge whether this could be justified in ethical terms. An alternative view of the situation would have been for the nurse to explain her reluctance to undertake advocacy on clinical grounds, but then to leave the final choice to the patient. If the patient was adamant that she wanted to go home, the nurse could have fulfilled her advocacy role by telling the doctors the woman's views, or by enabling the woman to speak up for herself. In either case, the nurse could still have told the doctors about her own reasons for opposing discharge. In this way she could have reconciled her duty as an advocate with her duty to safeguard the patient. It may be that this was indeed the fallback position that this nurse would have adopted if the patient had not accepted her initial recommendation to stay in hospital.

The issue of risk

The next step in Fig. 4.1 is probably the most neglected question of all: are you willing to risk advocacy? Many potential advocacy situations are highly emotive and it is easy for advocates to get carried away and identify so closely with their clients that they neglect to consider themselves. The examples in earlier chapters have already demonstrated that advocacy can be very risky, particularly for professionals who are employees of health care organisations. But even independent advocates need to consider the risks of damaged relationships, difficulties in gaining continued access to clients, or withdrawal of funding for their service, which may arise as consequences of advocacy on behalf of individuals. Further areas of risk to consider are those to the clients and those to colleagues in some situations. Because of the importance of this subject, a later chapter (Chapter 8) is devoted to risk and advocacy. At this point it is simply a matter of establishing that the question of risk management is part of most advocacy situations and is a legitimate consideration before commitments are made.

Self-advocacy or external advocacy?

If the risks have been identified and an advocacy approach accepted, Fig. 4.1 suggests that the next step is to consider whether, with help, the client can be enabled to self-advocate. This step therefore embodies a value judgement that self-advocacy is better than external advocacy. This judgement is in keeping with the emphasis on self-advocacy in the North American professional literature, where the main justification is that it lessens the risks to the helper. Of course it does not entirely eliminate risks. Anyone giving information or support to clients is likely to find that there will be some people in positions of authority who would prefer to see the information restricted and any support delivered by themselves alone. Nevertheless, the focus of attention is primarily on the client in self-advocacy and the helpers make less obvious targets than when they are acting as external advocates. A further source of support for self-advocacy comes from the experience of helpers in the fields of learning disabilities and mental health. To the extent that these clients can be helped to self-advocate successfully, the gains are twofold: the clients achieve their short term wants and they learn to become more independent of others than before. In contrast, successful external advocacy merely achieves the first short-term goal and in some situations it can make clients more dependent, since they learn that to get what they want they should enlist others to speak for them. Although these themes have been voiced most clearly in the areas of learning disabilities and mental health, they apply equally in all health care situations since they are strongly consistent with the emphasis on respect for autonomy and patients' rights which continues to grow in importance on both sides of the Atlantic.

Therefore it is argued that self-advocacy should be the preferred method of helping, all things being equal, because it promotes client autonomy and reduces the risks to helpers. However, as we know, all things are not always equal. Some clients have greater potential for self-advocacy than others; some situations demand technical knowledge, personal acquaintance or high level communication skills which can only be provided by an external advocate. The choice here is usually between independent advocates and health care professionals as advocates. Independent advocates provide a measure of independence and objectivity which is valuable to some clients and which makes them less vulnerable to retaliation from powerful people within the organisation. In contrast, health care professionals are more easily accessible by clients simply because of their numbers and patterns of work. Both types of external advocacy need to be considered in situations where self-advocacy is not possible or would stand a very limited chance of success. Bearing this in mind, each of the main decision points in Fig. 4.1 now needs to be examined, beginning in the next chapter with the initial assessment of wants.

Summary of key points

- Figure 4.1 can be used to clarify the decision-making process before helpers commit to advocacy
- The emphasis is on clients' wants rather than their needs
- Helpers may legitimately consider whether or not they can support clients' wants
- Advocacy risks should be identified in advance
- Self-advocacy should be the preferred method of helping, all other things being equal.

Chapter 5
Wants and Their Assessment

This chapter examines how clients express their wants and what those wants typically concern. The aim is to give some practical advice to both professional and independent advocates on how to assess, what to look for and what to avoid. It draws extensively on written examples of advocacy which were collected during a series of training courses. However, before looking at the detail of assessment, it is important to reiterate that the starting point for all forms of advocacy is what individuals 'want' as opposed to what they are thought to 'need'. This distinction places clients at the centre of the advocacy process. In contrast, the word 'need' carries the connotation of outsiders deciding what is right for clients. The distinction is similar to one made in counselling by Nelson Jones (1989) when he argued that counsellors should try to get in touch with the internal frame of reference of their clients, rather than forming judgements from an external frame of reference. Of course in advocacy the situation is complicated when clients are silent and their wants have to be ascribed to them, but even then an important difference emerges between weighing the evidence about their preferences in order to work out what silent clients want, as opposed to forming a judgement which uses only one's own experience as the basis for deciding what they need.

How clients express their wants

The pre-requisite for assessment is noticing things, being sensitive to the emotional state of particular individuals. The emotions which frequently give rise to the expression of wants are the unpleasant ones, particularly fear, anger and sorrow. We use a wide variety of words to try to capture the range of feelings within each of these emotional states, thinking most commonly in terms such as anxiety, worry, concern, nervousness, uncertainty, and different degrees of pain, discomfort or distress. These unpleasant and undesirable feelings may be stated directly in words by the individuals who are suffering them, or they may leak out in the form of non-verbal signs or particular types of behaviour. In some cases advocates are alerted to them by other people, such as clients' relatives or friends. In other cases the advocates infer particular feelings from what they know of their clients' situation as a form of empathy: 'If I were in that situation I would feel anxious, worried etc., so I assume that is how my client is feeling.' In practice people who are experiencing strong emotions tend to express these in several different ways at once. A description from an interview with a nurse on a surgical ward brings this out:

NURSE: 'The situation that sticks in my mind was a chap who was going to have major surgery to his face next day. He was very anxious because it was quite disfiguring and he was obviously concerned about what he was going to look like, how it was going to feel afterwards, how other people were going to react to him, and what effect it was going to have on his future. He became quite angry. He was off-ish with the rest of the staff.'

INTERVIEWER: 'And how did you first become aware that he was feeling angry or feeling off-ish?'

NURSE: 'Because we went in fairly regularly before he went to theatre to talk to him and the responses we got were abrupt. Silly things like meals weren't right, or the tea was cold when it obviously wasn't. Things like that. Expecting things to be done right away.'

INTERVIEWER: 'Were you aware then, when he was being angry and off-ish, of the reason for his worry, or not?'

NURSE: 'I went and spent some time with him. I sat down and said, "Are you worried about what is going to happen?" We then got on to the fact that he was worried and he wasn't sure whether to go ahead with the surgery or not. It was because he was scared that he was behaving this way. He said, "The consultant's spoken to me but I still don't understand it all properly." And I held his hand, let him have a cry. I think the physical contact was very important because he'd set up a big barrier around himself. I tried to be as honest and as open as possible about the surgery. I mean, there's no point pulling any punches about something like that. You can't soften the blow, though I wasn't unkind either.'

INTERVIEWER: 'What would have happened if you hadn't, if you'd sort of minimised it?'

NURSE: 'I think that we would have lost a friend really. Because we did become quite close, all of the staff. And I think he would have felt betrayed if we'd lied to him.'

So the want which this patient was expressing was a want for more information to enable him to decide whether to go ahead with the proposed operation. The patient had given initial consent at an out-patient appointment with the consultant and had signalled continuing consent by allowing himself to be admitted to the hospital. However, as the time of the operation drew closer, his anxiety and uncertainty about the consequences of major facial surgery became stronger and stronger. Initially his feelings were expressed obliquely in words and behaviour which were unusually sharp for him. The nurse had to be alert to the meaning of this change in behaviour and to see beyond it to the underlying cause, perhaps even before the patient was consciously aware of it himself. The nurse made an empathic inference that the patient wanted more information about the consequences of the operation, but then took care to confirm this in conversation. Once the patient realised the nurse was prepared to get emotionally close to him and listen, then he felt able to express his wants very clearly in words. In this case the nurse empowered the patient with additional information, which helped him to make his own choice to go ahead with the surgery. The lessons to be drawn are that emotions tend to come to the surface ahead of their verbal expression; that helpers sometimes need to watch for unusual behaviour and infer the deeper meaning; and that advocates frequently have to get emotionally close to their clients in order to enable them to feel safe enough to express their wants.

Identifying strength of feeling

When trying to help clients who have the capacity to say what they want, it is particularly important to assess their wishes carefully, including the strength of those wishes. The reason is that some clients may say that they want one thing and the advocate speaks up on their behalf, but then they change their minds. Sometimes this is deliberately manipulative, but more usually it means that the initial want was not especially strong or clear in the person's own mind. Sometimes also the helpers decide what clients need and then try to convince the clients that this is what they really want. Another example from a surgical ward illustrates the problems:

'This particular patient was due in theatre later on the shift for an investigative operation. In the past he'd had some other major operations and each time had complications from them including chest infections and a cardiac arrest. I talked to the patient beforehand and he asked me about the pros and cons. I gave him the information as best I could and he said that he would prefer to postpone the operation until his general health improved. I thought this was a good decision and assured him that he had every right to make this clear when the doctor came down. But when the anaesthetist visited to get the consent he saw the patient on his own and, by the time he left, the patient had agreed to have the surgery as scheduled. I questioned the anaesthetist about it and pointed out the patient's history and that he had said to me he wanted to postpone the operation. I felt the patient had not been fully informed about all the possible risks and may have been forced into agreeing. The anaesthetist was not willing to admit this and the surgical team would not intervene. I went back to the patient and asked him what had happened. He told me he had not been pressurised into changing his mind but that he had been persuaded. He said he was happy to go ahead and have the operation. Some time later a junior member of staff told me the patient had said he felt the anaesthetist had made the decision for him. I spoke with my manager but we decided there was nothing more we could do.'

Here the patient was fully autonomous and clearly expressed his wants. The difficulty is that he did so at least twice and said different things to different people! There is no reason to believe that the patient was being deliberately manipulative as he had no real interest in being so. The question turns on whether he was permitted to give voluntary and informed consent to the operation. When the nurse heard that he had consented to the operation, she assumed the role of advocate and questioned the anaesthetist before checking her mandate with the patient. This appears to have been a mistake, because when she did eventually ask the patient he said he had changed his mind willingly, thus completely undermining her position. Although the patient later told someone else he felt he had been forced to change his mind by the anaesthetist, the nurse no longer felt able to take on an advocacy role in case the patient withdrew his support yet again. It is easy to be wise after the event, but in this situation the nurse needed not only to identify the patient's concerns but also to get the patient to be explicit about what he wanted from her. Did he want the nurse to support him in calling back the anaesthetist, or to speak out on his behalf, or simply to do nothing?

Contrast that example with one given by a district nurse who was visiting a woman in her own home soon after a mastectomy operation when she was awaiting a follow-up appointment with the consultant:

'Mary is a young woman who wants to get on with her life. She desperately needs to know the way forward, but she was beginning to withdraw into herself and away from her family. On some visits she had bouts of intense euphoria but these were followed by bouts of depression during which she retired to her bedroom away from her family. She related how after finding the lump she was told "It will be all

right". She went into hospital – "it will be all right". She had the mastectomy – "it will be all right". She was learning to live with her disfigurement but couldn't cope with running to the letterbox every day
only to find no appointment letter had arrived and she didn't know if she
needed chemotherapy or radiotherapy. She said she was really worried about seeing the consultant without support. Her husband is
another "it'll be all right" sort of guy. She is extremely tired of "it'll be all
right". So having heard all this I asked her what she wanted to happen.
She said she really hoped the consultant would give her the all-clear
but when I pressed her she said, "I want to know the truth – no lying. I
want my appointment and someone I can trust to be with me during it."
I asked her, "What if the truth isn't what you want to hear?" She said,
"Be it good or bad I need to plan for the future." Finally I asked her if
she had heard of the Macmillan nurses and did she know their role. I
asked if she would be willing to meet one of them and see if they were
the right person to go with her to the appointment and she agreed.'

The district nurse went on to say that she asked the patient to write
down all the questions she wanted to ask the consultant. The Macmillan
nurse visited, speeded up the appointment and attended with the
patient. In order to reach this outcome, the precise questioning by the
district nurse was vital in enabling her to go beyond an on-the-surface
statement of the client's wants to explore the true strength of those
wants and what would need to happen to fulfil them.

Silent clients

Ideally an assessment should include an explicit and agreed mandate
from clients for the type of advocacy to be undertaken. An obvious
problem here is what to do when clients are silent – are there rational
ways of identifying the wants of silent clients? As elsewhere in this book,
it is useful to begin with an example and then to discuss the issue using
the clinical situation as a starting point. This one was provided by an
enrolled nurse working in a medical ward with a seriously ill and literally
silent patient:

'The problem was lack of nutritional intake. The patient was in danger
of starvation and was unable to speak or swallow. The consultant said
that a naso-gastric tube should be passed urgently. A nurse on the
ward explained the procedure to the patient, stating that it may be
uncomfortable and to try to gulp to help the tube pass easier. There
was a bewildered look on the patient's face. The nurse proceeded to
pass the tube but the patient retched and took out the tube. The nurse

attempted the procedure again but when the tube was put to the patient's nostril she became distressed, flapping a hand and turned her head away. I told the nurse the patient was distressed and not to try again as she was non-verbally saying she didn't want it. The nurse ignored my advice, saying she daren't disobey the consultant. I told her I would have a word with the registrar. He spoke to the consultant and to the patient and relatives. A peg tube was advised and accepted, so the patient received nutrition and fluids.'

There can be little doubt based on this account that the enrolled nurse correctly interpreted the patients' wants when she spoke up on her behalf. The non-verbal evidence of the patient's distress was compelling and obvious. The consultant later expanded on this assessment by speaking to the relatives, who were able to reaffirm the meaning of the patient's non-verbal behaviour. In this case their independence, as well as the independent spirit of the enrolled nurse, helped to safeguard the patient. At the very least some form of independent confirmation of one's interpretation of a silent patient's wants is desirable whenever possible. However, in situations or at times when consultation is not possible, a helper may still combine knowledge and experience with careful observation to infer the patient's wants, as in the situation described below:

'My patient was dying of acute myeloid leukaemia. The doctors were continuing with chemotherapy. The patient was in a great deal of pain. A diamorphine pump was in situ but was not as effective as it could have been. Oramorph was prescribed but was not given by the other nurses on the ward as the patient was semi-conscious and thrashing around. I called for the doctor who said she would come when she was not too busy. After a while she had not arrived so I called again. I should have left the ward at the end of my shift but I was concerned about the patient's condition. I continued to call the senior house officer (SHO) at intervals of ten minutes until she arrived. This was about 10:15pm. The SHO said that she would increase the diamorphine pump infusion and strength when the pump needed changing. I knew this would not be until 2pm the next day. I then, with force, asked the doctor to look at the patient and see her father, brother, etc. and then asked if she would like to see any of her relatives in this condition and asked her what she would do to relieve their suffering.

My reasons for taking this blunt action were because I put myself into my patient's and his family's shoes. I was able to do this easily because the same thing had happened to me with one of my relatives, therefore I understood the distress the situation put the family in. The only risks were upsetting the SHO and, as I knew my reasons were correct, I did not worry. Other options were to call the SHO's superior or the sister on call. I decided not to take this alternative because I felt that I could make the SHO understand the need for prompt action. The SHO increased the dosage in the pump right away and also gave him an injection of haloperidol. This aided my patient's breathing and helped him to have a peaceful and dignified death. I believe my intervention was successful as the family felt less anxious when the time came and their distress and the patient's distress eased.'

The emotional involvement of the nurse with *her* patient comes across very strongly. She believed that she was in touch with what the patient would have wanted had he been in any condition to voice his wants. She also had the technical knowledge about medication to know what would or would not be effective in this situation. Finally she had the confidence to insist on the junior doctor attending and to persist in trying to persuade the doctor to see what was so obvious to the nurse herself, that the patient needed help immediately. This is the kind of situation where a professional advocate can be particularly effective, combining knowledge of the patient with technical knowledge of health care issues. Some discussion with colleagues or with the relatives to check on their support might have been advisable, but in the end who can gainsay the actions of this powerful advocate?

The issues facing clients

Effective advocates need to have an understanding of the main issues which they are likely to uncover when assessing clients. There is a long literature on the vast range of anxieties and fears experienced by all types of clients in contact with health care services (see for example Hayward 1975; Miles 1984; Thorne & Robinson 1988; Wilson-Barnett & Carrigy 1978). In a research study which involved tape recorded interviews with patients I found that, despite great variety in the detail, the overall set of issues could be described using fairly predictable categories such as concerns about health, treatments, the environment of care, and relatives and other loved ones (Teasdale 1992b).

Health

It is hardly surprising that concerns about state of health figured strongly in both hospital and community settings. The nature of the concerns depended on the stage patients had reached in their contact with professional help. They ranged from initial uncertainty about diagnosis, through to concerns about prognosis and in some cases to the final certainty of death. Uncertainty appeared to be a major problem for patients. Aside from worries about life, death and disability, some patients found it hard to cope with the loss of control which arose from their contact with the health care services. A woman who had to have a mastectomy following discovery of a breast lump, at a routine check-up graphically described her feelings:

> 'And here of course I'm not in control. I mean, I went for an insurance medical five weeks ago and the doctor found the lump . . . And things just came to a stop. Again I wasn't in control. And as I said to the doctor, "Fifteen days ago I didn't have a problem. You doctors created the problem".'

Treatments

An area where the majority of patients seem to feel deprived of information concerns worries about different types of treatments. Surgery is a treatment which may be routine to many of the professionals but which is anything but routine to most of the patients. Patients who were interviewed were anxious about dying while under anaesthetic, about the surgeon making a mistake, about pain during or after the operation, and about the disfiguring consequences of some treatments. However, they also reported concerns about treatments other than surgery, including many aspects of nursing care. Examples included fears about pain during investigative procedures, concerns over catching AIDS from blood transfusions, worries about different types of rehabilitation procedure, anxiety about the desensitisation treatments used by psychologists, and concerns about medication. In many cases there is a painful tension between hope of recovery and fear of the treatment, which may inhibit information seeking, with individuals preferring to concentrate their minds on their hopes rather than on their fears.

Many patients feel that they have no real choice or control over treatment and therefore see no value in empowerment or advocacy. The problem is that in serious disease the choice of treatment is very limited and comes down to accepting a frightening intervention or suffering the consequences of the disease. Many patients regard this as no choice at all. In addition, decisions about treatment are sometimes taken without the full agreement of the patient. This seems to happen particularly frequently to people who can be stereotyped as not fully autonomous, for example elderly people who appear disorientated by hospital admission or people with learning disabilities who are admitted without specialist helpers or relatives at their side. Thus a nurse reported finding an elderly patient anxious about a change of medication:

> 'When I asked her why she was upset she said it was because the doctor had taken her off her steroids without any discussion because he said they would "poison your system". She had been taking them for five years for her rheumatoid arthritis and knew what it was like without them, so she didn't mind "poisoning" herself, as they helped.'

In this case the nurse acted as advocate for the patient and persuaded the doctor to restore the steroid medication.

The environment of care

People in their own homes can control the environment when professionals come to visit. In hospital the environment of care is controlled by others and many patients see it as an alien and disempowering place. Newly hospitalised patients can be troubled by their dependence on others in aspects of everyday living hitherto taken for granted, such as being unable to find their way to the toilet or bathroom, not knowing how to summon help when required or being unsure of the hospital routine and rules. Patients who are vulnerable by reason of age or disability tend to regard any change in their environment with particular trepidation:

> 'The patient was slightly mentally handicapped and I don't think she really understood what was happening to her. She was frightened of the new surroundings and probably of the people she did not know.'

> 'He (a four year old boy) was worried about being placed in an unfamiliar environment with lots of strange faces. He was being removed from his mother and brothers and sisters. During the first few hours he was consistently tearful and cried out for his mother. He also refused to accept that he had to stay in hospital and said that he would be going home as soon as he'd had his dinner.'

Many hospitalised patients have concerns about their possessions, either those left at home or the safety of money or jewellery they had brought into hospital with them. In the former case, elderly people have particular problems when their disabilities lead to them moving from their own homes into nursing homes and the move is organised by others while they are still hospitalised. People with short-term memory loss are also particularly vulnerable to worries about possessions:

'The patient was wandering up and down the ward talking to other patients and searching in cupboards and on shelves . . . I approached him and talked with him and he sounded very anxious. At the time I presumed that the patient had lost something. He had poor short-term memory and had often mislaid things in the past.'

The nurse noted the tendency of this patient to misplace his possessions and then even to forget what he was searching for. This type of situation presents particular problems to helpers who are trying to assess the nature of the concerns of essentially silent patients. Prior knowledge of the individual is clearly important and supports the arguments of independent advocates that a long-term advocacy relationship is highly desirable.

Concerns about relatives and other loved ones

For many people illness comes as an interruption to an everyday life in which they are more used to caring for others than being cared for themselves. For example, an elderly patient who was admitted for a total hip replacement became very irritable and made himself unpopular with the staff:

'He seemed very agitated and distracted. No one seemed to have much time or sympathy and he was often aggressive and abusive. I thought he was anxious about his wife as they both lived at home with each other, had no children, and he looked after her. So while he was in hospital she had been taken to a nursing home. He continually asked about her and wanted to know how long it would be before he could go home as he wanted to see his wife, as he said they didn't have many years left and they wanted to spend what little time they had left together.'

The nurse acted as advocate for the patient with the other staff and also facilitated telephone contact with the patient's wife while he was in hospital. It was important that the nurse had a hunch about the cause of the patient's irritable behaviour, since this had isolated him from the majority of the staff. In this case the patient's physical state had interfered with his ability to continue everyday life as usual.

However, for some psychiatric patients the position is reversed, with everyday worries about family or friends forming the very subject of the problems which bring them into contact with health care services:

'Well, I lost my daughter-in-law when she was 26 in a very bad accident. Now the two children, they're ten and eight, and they've been with my daughter, they've been with her two years. But it's suddenly come into my mind, "What if she didn't want them any more?" She's promised faithfully that she will keep them. And I know, but it's making my brain accept it. And I was getting myself down, getting everybody down, but they were very kind and listened. It was only a small thing but to me it was a mountain.'

As well as worrying about other people, pets also figure in the concerns of many hospitalised patients. Animals can be very important as companions, particularly to isolated elderly people, and the distress the patients suffer as a result of separation from their pets during hospitalisation is the same as if their companions were human. A nurse described a typical incident where an elderly woman became very anxious on admission:

'Her background was that she had been living alone and her home situation was getting worse. And she had a little dog, and a lot of the time she was actually running round the ward trying to find her dog. And she was getting more and more anxious, and of course the dog wasn't there. I think initially for the first week or so it was quite good if you just stayed with her and said the dog was with her next-door neighbour, which it was. And that the dog was being looked after. The problem was that she was wanting to go home, but her home was being sold and she was waiting for a placement in a nursing home.'

This situation had a happy ending with the nurse intervening to bring the dog to the hospital for a visit and also ensuring that the nursing home chosen would accept the dog when the woman was discharged. However, the same nurse described another case in which a patient's dog was destroyed while he was in hospital because the neighbours were unable to look after it. A linking theme between both situations is the way decisions were made without consulting the patients, leaving them uncertain about the fate of their pets and distressed at their own inability to exercise any control over what was happening.

Clearly there is enormous scope for advocacy in all these situations, where patients will want information to reduce uncertainty and opportunities to exercise some degree of control over events or to prevent even greater losses in this area. It can be seen that assessment requires high level observation and empathic skills, plus in depth knowledge of the system and the options realistically available to patient. This needs to be accompanied by sensitivity to the variations in the strength of the concerns of individuals and their capacity for self advocacy through empowerment.

Summary of key points

- Assessment of wants is a task that takes time and care to complete
- Non-verbal signs and out-of-character behaviour frequently provide cues
- Strength of feeling needs to be established
- Where patients are silent, it is useful to discuss ascribed wants with objective others
- Patients' concerns tend to fall under four headings:

  (1) Health
  (2) Treatments
  (3) The environment of care
  (4) Concerns about relatives and other loved ones

- Two threads link patients' concerns: uncertainty about the future and a perceived lack of control over events
- Those patients who are not regarded as fully autonomous by their carers are particularly vulnerable to being deprived of control over events.

Chapter 6
Empowering Clients to Self-Advocate

Empowerment means giving information or support to individuals to help them to undertake self-advocacy. It contrasts with external advocacy, which involves helpers speaking up on behalf of clients. In order to empower other people we have to start with a belief that they are capable of making informed choices for themselves, that they are autonomous individuals. However, autonomy is not an all-or-nothing concept. There are degrees of autonomy. For example, a person suffering from a psychotic illness such as schizophrenia will experience disturbances in rational thinking, but these may fluctuate over time or may affect only limited areas of the person's functioning. Thus some individuals learn about their illness and can choose the type of help or support that they need when their rational thinking abilities begin to deteriorate. In the same way, some sick children aged five years or even younger will have the mental capacity to appreciate basic treatment choices, whereas others will not have developed sufficient maturity. Therefore helpers need to judge the degree of autonomy of their clients before they decide whether or not to use empowerment.

Unfortunately this judgement is sometimes related to the outcomes of the decision-making process. Typically this means that if a patient agrees with the course of treatment recommended by the professionals, the patient is deemed to be autonomous, whereas if the recommended line is rejected this is taken as proof that the patient lacks the capacity to make an informed choice. As Beauchamp & Childress (1979) point out, this approach cannot be justified in ethical terms. To abide by the moral principle of respect for autonomy, any judgement about mental capacity must be made *before* choices are offered and the helpers must be prepared in advance to accept the outcomes, even where they differ from their own views. In order to avoid the charge of paternalism, it is necessary also to start with the presumption that an individual is capable of acting autonomously unless evidence to the contrary is forthcoming. This idea also supports the preference in Fig. 4.1 for self-advocacy over external advocacy, when all other things are equal. Professionals are particularly vulnerable to slipping into paternalism when their motivation is to do good for patients and they believe that their knowledge and experience are so great that they can predict outcomes with a high degree of certainty. Independent advocates have an advantage in these situations because they are not involved in giving treatment to their clients and so can maintain an objectivity which the professionals sometimes find elusive.

John Southgate (1988) is a writer with a psychoanalytical background who sees five aspects to advocacy based on empowerment:

(1) Nurturing
(2) Being a witness
(3) Protesting against what has been done
(4) Translating what has happened
(5) Supporting the client's inner child.

These five aspects emphasise the emotional closeness which empowering approaches may require to convince what Kate White (1990) describes as our 'little caretaker self' that it is safe to relax and express genuine feelings in the presence of a sensitive and caring advocate. These concerns with the emotional wellbeing of clients are important, because they spell out the support function of this type of advocacy and so help to balance the usual emphasis on straightforward information-giving. In a research study of the nursing management of anxious patients, personal support interventions were found to be particularly valued by hospitalised patients (Teasdale 1995).

Systematic empowerment

A valuable analysis of empowerment has been given by Sheila Corcoran (1994) in which she links Gadow's (1980b) model of ethical decision-making with the idea of using a decision tree to decide what information should be collected by a helper. Corcoran explains that Gadow's ideas about empowering patients go beyond simple information-giving. Gadow argues that helpers need to assist patients not only in acquiring information but also in analysing what they want for themselves, based on their personal values and beliefs. This involves the helpers in getting emotionally close to patients, echoing the approach of Southgate (1988) and White (1990).

Gadow (1980b) proposed five steps for promoting patient involvement in decision-making, looking from the perspective of a nurse or other professional helper:

(1) Ensuring that the patient has relevant information
(2) Enabling the patient to select information
(3) Disclosing the helper's own views
(4) Helping the patient to determine personal values
(5) Helping the patient determine the meaning of any choices made.

Corcoran (1994) illustrated these ideas through a case study of a woman experiencing the menopause and facing a decision about oestrogen replacement therapy. In step one, the nurse identified three options open to the patient: to take oestrogen on its own, to take a combination therapy, or to take no hormones at all. She also considered the risks and possible outcomes associated with each option. In step two, the nurse briefly described the types of information others had found useful and added that she was willing to share her own views and preferences if the patient thought this would help. The patient indicated that initially she would like to know about the options open to her, explaining that she was worried about her menopausal symptoms and knew there was a family history of osteoporosis. The nurse drew a simplified decision tree showing the possibility that taking oestrogen might restore hormonal balance but also the possibility that a balance might be hard to achieve. Beyond these possibilities, the decision tree also included branches showing the chances of osteoporosis or of no osteoporosis, and of endometrial cancer or no cancer. The nurse consulted with the gynaecologist and gave rough estimates of the probabilities of the different outcomes. The nurse was careful to respond to what the patient wanted and not to force information onto the patient. After considering the decision tree, the patient asked the nurse what she would do in her situation. The nurse responded, giving her own personal view. Corcoran argues that this is only appropriate if the patient indicates that such information would be useful. She also cautions that,

'The nurse should recognise nurses' and patients' unequal positions of power within the typical health care bureaucracy. Nurses' values and opinions shared from a relative position of power may have persuasive or even coercive force, despite the intent. Therefore the manner in which such information is communicated can make a significant difference in whether the patient perceives it as additional information and an invitation to explore values, or as an attempt to persuade' (Corcoran 1994, p.161).

In the case study the patient then went over her doubts and concerns, but said that the information had helped her and she would probably choose a combined therapy, although she would take a bit more time to be sure. Finally the nurse discussed the personal meaning of the menopause for this particular patient and how the decision to accept hormone replacement fitted in with her values and beliefs. Corcoran offered this combination of ideas from Gadow (1980b) and from decision theory (Corcoran 1986) as a guide to encourage helpers to explore new ways of aiding patients to make decisions. Clearly the five steps are valuable for any helper who wants to reflect on empowerment in practice, although the use of a written decision tree may appear unduly complicated and time consuming in everyday clinical practice. In fact when comparing actual clinical examples I have collected with Corcoran's theoretical case study, there are none as comprehensive and systematic as Corcoran's example. This presents a problem. Are British helpers failing their clients by not being sufficiently systematic in their use of empowerment, or can effective empowerment take place without going to the lengths described by Corcoran?

The following example from an interview with the nurse in charge of a breast cancer clinic brings out some of the issues:

'The patient came out of the clinic to look for me. I'd counselled her when she first found out she had breast cancer, so she just came to my office and said, "Can I have a few words". She told me she was very upset because the doctor had recommended a change of treatment. He had said, "I think it might be better if you had a mastectomy, because of possible local recurrence." And when she had raised objections to this, he'd agreed that he would do radiotherapy. After she'd had time to think about it she realised she maybe was putting her life at risk by going against, or thinking she was going against, his recommendation. And she wanted to talk it over.'

In this situation the patient had made a choice already, but was now having second thoughts about it. Having raised treatment options with the doctor, she had been given some information about these, although we are not told what or how much. The nurse went on to supply some additional information:

'So we discussed it for a little while and I explained to her why he probably said that, in view of the fact that she'd already had some spread to the axilla and he was afraid that there would be some secondary deposits in the breast already. And that was probably what he was saying it for. That he didn't want her to have to come back and have a mastectomy in another six months or a year. And I also said to her that he was very unlikely to agree to radiotherapy if he felt he was putting her at risk. The only risk I felt that she was bringing to light was the risk of having to have the mastectomy at some later date and this was a lot higher risk than the normal person would have.'

Here the nurse was drawing on her knowledge of the consultant's general treatment policies with the effect of supporting the choice that the patient had made. It appears that the nurse was selecting information for the patient and presenting it to her, rather than encouraging her to identify her information needs for herself, as Corcoran and Gadow suggest. The nurse in the example avoided talking about outcomes, although she did deal at a general level with the likelihood of the patient having to have a mastectomy at a later date even if she rejected it now – which is in line with Corcoran's advice about probabilities. It is unclear how much the nurse was responding to specific requests made by the patient and how much she was volunteering what she thought was relevant.

The nurse went on to offer to check her interpretation, but the consultant had already left. However she and the registrar examined the notes. They considered that the cancer had probably already spread to other parts of the breast so there was a very high chance that the patient would have to have a mastectomy in the end. However the registrar supported the nurse's view that the consultant would not have agreed to begin with radiotherapy alone if he felt it would put the patient's life at risk. The nurse then returned and said, 'Well really what I've said is the way it's been'. It appears therefore that the nurse was limiting the detail of the information she was prepared to give to the patient and addressing only the original question asked, about whether the patient's preference for radiotherapy alone would put her life at risk. In the event, the patient asked the nurse if she could come back the next afternoon to talk it over again with her husband present. The nurse described this second interview:

'So when she came back with her husband she said he was behind her decision one hundred per cent, but they still wanted it explaining in detail. And because they're a very sensible pair, I thought it important I gave them a bit more information than I would perhaps give to the average couple. So I explained that we had no way of knowing whether there had already been spread beyond the axilla. So whichever decision on treatment she made, it wouldn't be her fault if suddenly we had to give her some treatment for a secondary elsewhere. That rather pleased her, surprisingly. So I said really the only thing was that she'd got to face up to the very strong possibility that sometime or other she would have to have a mastectomy if a local recurrence occurred. But we would check regularly if this was happening. So she's gone off quite happy about it now. But I did think it was important, it was a judgement. I wouldn't normally talk ... I mean everyone talks about secondaries, you need to let them realise that this is the accepted thing, you just have to look after them and treat them. But I thought in her case it was important for her to know that any secondary that came, if ever, wouldn't be as a result of the action she was taking this time. But she certainly wasn't in a position to accept a mastectomy.'

As far as one can judge the nurse appears to have staged the disclosure of risks over the two interviews. In the first one she presented information which supported the patient's choice, emphasising that the consultant would have argued the case for a mastectomy much more strongly if he really believed there was immediate danger. In the second interview, and with the patient supported by her husband, the nurse went further and disclosed some of the information that she had acquired from her review of the case notes with the registrar, namely that a mastectomy was likely to be necessary at some time in the future. This approach appears to be much less open than that of the nurse in the imaginary example described by Corcoran. However, the outpatients nurse appeared to have a very close relationship with the patient as is confirmed by the way the patient reacted to her. She went on to say that at one point the patient asked what symptoms of secondaries she should look for.

'I said, "I'm not going to tell you because you'll dream them up if I do." I said, "No worry, we will be looking for the symptoms, we will be doing the checks." She said, "I'm glad you didn't tell me because I would have worried".'

Is this paternalism or empathic understanding? I am inclined to support the nurse's actions, particularly because of how she went on to summarise her overall view of what the patient wanted:

'She desperately needed not to have somebody take the decision for her, but to know that any future developments wouldn't be as a result of the decision she was making now... She asked me what I would do and I said, "I can't say what I would do because I'm not in your situation. But I would do what I would feel happiest doing." I always use this tack. Whilst you've got a choice, because the consultants are giving a choice all the time – virtually every patient's given a choice. I usually give a little warning if he would prefer the choice was in one direction. I would probably tend to overplay the good side of that particular treatment, if he's made it clear to me that that's really what he wants to do. But advice, no. It's not a good idea. Facts and reassurance... The only advice I'd give is, "Think about it. Sooner or later it will come to light, what you really want to do, what you feel happiest doing".'

It seems to me that this is a sensitive, empowering approach based around a close and trusting relationship with patients and a philosophy which emphasises the right to choose. The consultants at this particular clinic appear to have allowed this nurse genuine freedom to act as an empowering counsellor to patients. She is a member of the team and therefore knows their own preferences, but these are not imposed on the patients. This approach seems to be in keeping with the underlying philosophy of Gadow (1980b) and Corcoran (1994) based on a trusting relationship and respect for the patient's autonomy, but with the detail adapted to the realities of everyday clinical practice.

Prediction and control

One of the greatest problems for patients and helpers that the preceding example brings out is how to manage uncertainty, particularly uncertainty associated with treatment choices and health outcomes. Suzanne Miller (1979) has explored these issues and found that there are two types of information which can be given to patients:

(1)   Predictive information
(2)   Information for control.

Predictive information tells patients what is going to happen in terms of their health and related treatment. This is very much the type of information which the out-patients nurse was giving and which she referred to as 'facts and reassurance'. In contrast, information for control allows an individual to influence the outcome of events and is often sought by patients. Miller proposed the 'minimax' hypothesis as a theoretical explanation of the relationship between controllability and human stress. Minimax states that:

'Individuals are motivated by a desire to minimise the maximum danger to themselves. Therefore they prefer and are less stressed by control, when having control allows them to put an upper limit on how bad the situation can become.' (Miller *et al.* 1989, p.108)

According to Miller there are three types of control:

(1)   Avoidance of an unwelcome event
(2)   Escape from an unwelcome event that has already commenced
(3)   Mitigation of the things that make the event unwelcome.

Most of the control offered by helpers to patients is of the mitigation variety, for example letting patients self-administer pain killing tablets when they want them, or choosing between different types of anaesthetic before an operation. The out-patients example was a rare instance of avoidance of an unwelcome mastectomy, at least for a limited period of time. Examples of escape would be giving information that allowed patients to exercise their right to discharge themselves or to withdraw consent to an operation at the last moment. One of the problems for professionals, particularly those working in the increasingly hi-tech world of modern medical and surgical care, is that the opportunities for patients to exercise meaningful control over events are limited by the overawing effect of the technology and of the complex patient-processing systems of the organisations which administer treatments. Both tend to make patients compliant and unaware of their right to question what is being done to them. Also the sheer pressure of numbers and cost consciousness have led to a culture, particularly in hospitals, where for many aspects of treatment and care consent is assumed unless forcefully indicated to the contrary. The usual indication of a possible withdrawal of consent is when a patient shows signs of anxiety or stress in the face of an impending treatment. In this situation there is a strong tendency for the professional helpers to use information predictive of a safe outcome to reassure and so pacify patients, rather than to encourage patients to exercise control over events. Two examples will make this distinction clear:

'One morning on a doctor's round the patient was told that a place had become available at an old people's nursing home and that she would be going sometime next week. It had been discussed with her about two months previously and her relatives had chosen that particular nursing home... Obviously she was worried about leaving hospital and going to a strange new home. She did not want to leave... We explained why she was going to the new nursing home and talked about what it would be like – they go on outings, play bingo and watch television. She was taken by her relatives to see it (didn't really work – she hated the place at first sight). Her relatives encouraged her by saying it was closer and that they could visit more often. Before she left a big effort was made to get her a new dress and make her look as she wished. Opportunity was given for her to talk about the new home. Another patient was to go there the next week so she was introduced to him.'

In this first example the patient is given plenty of information about the new nursing home, but it has nothing to do with empowerment. The information is almost entirely predictive and designed to reassure the patient and increase her compliance. The only control permitted seems to have been over the purchase of a new dress. The decision about a nursing home was taken two months previously and the patient's evident lack of consent to the move appears to have been ignored by both professionals and relatives. This is precisely the type of situation where independent advocacy is needed. A contrasting example involves an 85 year old woman who was living in her own home and who contacted a district nurse:

'The next day when visiting Mrs X I chatted for a few minutes about the weather etc. and then asked her how I could help, as I could see she was "jumpy". The problem was decreased mobility which meant she couldn't manage the stairs very well. This led on to me asking her about problems with getting on and off the toilet, in and out of the bath, and managing housework. I told her that help was available in the form of aids and appliances and we discussed the advantage of having the bed downstairs. She was against this as she only had a double bed, but when I said she could apply for financial help as she was on supplementary benefit she thought this was a good idea. I then suggested that she might apply to housing for a sheltered flat which would solve many problems, but realised that this suggestion upset her as she and her husband had worked to buy the house for many years. Therefore I did not pursue this idea. I did a follow-up visit two weeks after the initial visit. Mrs X was much more relaxed as the social services had fitted her with bath and toilet aids and a commode which meant she didn't have to come downstairs during the night. She was quite happy about having a bed downstairs as she had heard that she had been given a grant towards a new bed and bedding. She had also decided not to pursue the idea of sheltered accommodation at the moment but promised that she would get in touch with me again if she changed her mind. She is going to ring me when the bed comes so that I can go and admire it!'

The information given by the district nurse allowed the woman to exercise real control over her environment by making her aware of the range of support to which she was entitled. The one contentious issue was the suggestion about sheltered accommodation. The nurse was sensitive enough to see that this was unacceptable, but one wonders whether part of the difference between this example and the previous one is that this woman was still living in her own home. Certainly analysis of the case studies which I have collected suggests that empowering interventions occur much more freely in community rather than in hospital settings. This may be connected with the philosophies and skills of professionals working in the community, but it seems likely that both professionals and patients are influenced by their working environment. In fact many professionals reveal their underlying thinking by reserving the term 'clients' for people living in their own homes and using 'patients' for those admitted to hospitals.

An overview of empowerment

In the sixteenth century Francis Bacon stated that 'knowledge itself is power'. This continues to hold true today, particularly in health care settings. Knowledge, or information as we prefer to call it, is the basis for all empowering interventions. However, it has to be information of a type that allows people to exercise meaningful control over their situation and not just information designed to reassure individuals into accepting the status quo. The Internet is beginning to make freely available information which used to be very hard to access (Teasdale & Teasdale 1996). There are websites associated with self-help organisations and particular forms of illness. There are also usergroups which allow individuals to post questions and then receive answers from any-one who chooses to reply. Recently when I was working with a focus group of cancer patients one member of the group revealed that she had posted questions about particular drug treatments which she was receiving and said that the answers she had received were far more informative than anything she had been told at the clinic. In contrast, professionals are under subtle pressures to restrict information for control based on concerns to use their time effectively and sometimes on a general approach which places a high value on protective, caring approaches (Malin & Teasdale 1991).

The antidote is a philosophy which emphasises the importance of respect for autonomy, together with careful analysis of the types of information which people need if they are to make choices and exercise control. Some groups of vulnerable people may still require the additional objectivity which independent advocacy schemes can offer. But no matter who is doing the empowering, it must also be based on a relationship of trust in which information is not forced on individuals but is freely available to them when they want it. In many respects non-directive counselling and empowerment are the same thing. As early as the 1950s Carl Rogers (1957) proposed that the foundations of a counselling relationship are empathy, warmth and genuineness. By empathy he meant an emotional closeness, seeing the world through the eyes of the client; by warmth he meant caring; and by genuineness he meant honesty. Non-directive counselling is intended to help clients decide things for themselves and as such Rogers' three characteristics may be seen as the basis of all forms of empowering relationships, as well as being relevant in external advocacy.

Summary of key points

- Empowerment means helping clients to self-advocate
- Theorists have argued that empowerment involves ensuring clients have relevant information, helping them to select what they want, disclosing the helper's own views on request, and helping clients to determine their personal values and the personal meaning of any choices they make
- In practice these ideas can guide helpers but appear to be too prescriptive to follow exactly in every situation
- The distinction between predictive information and information for control is important; only the latter is truly empowering
- Opportunities for clients to exercise control are more limited in hospital settings than in the community
- As well as giving information, empowerment also means supporting patients through establishing close emotional relationships which are based on the same values as non-directive counselling – empathy, warmth and genuineness.

Chapter 7
External Advocacy

This chapter concentrates on situations where helpers plead for or defend clients who are unable or unwilling to do this for themselves. This form of advocacy involves what Mallik (1997) describes as a triadic relationship, with the three parties being the client, the advocate and at least one other person who has the authority to grant or refuse what the advocate wants. The process of undertaking advocacy in these circumstances may be divided into three steps:

(1) Agreeing a contract with the client
(2) Planning for external advocacy
(3) Presenting the client's case.

In practice these three steps may overlap. In emergency situations the move from agreeing a contract through to presenting a case may leave little or no time for preparation. When working with a patient who is unconscious, or for other reasons unable to express wants, the contract will be assumed rather than agreed. Presentation of the patient's case may be a shared enterprise involving the patient or relatives, with the advocate taking more of a background and supportive role. However, the three steps are useful in teasing out the process of external advocacy in health care and in making links with other concepts which can cast light on advocacy practice. Therefore this chapter begins by discussing each step in turn, but includes a variety of case studies that go behind the three steps to illustrate the complex reality of everyday advocacy.

Agreeing a contract

An advocacy contract should clearly specify what the client wants and how strongly those wants are felt. It is essential that the advocate is sympathetic to the client's concerns, or at the very least supports the client's right to have those concerns expressed to others. The advocate must be clear about whose wants are being represented and must be able to justify the choice of external advocacy over self-advocacy. Finally, the ideal contract specifies how the advocacy will be undertaken and at what point the advocate will consult further with the client. A situation described by a health visitor illustrates the main points:

> 'An 11 year old boy was referred to me by a school nurse. He had a bed-wetting problem and had sought advice and help from the GP without any resolution of the problem. The GP would only prescribe one type of treatment, which had failed, and was unwilling to consider others or further referral. The boy was very anxious to become dry. I spoke to his mother who backed up everything he had told me. She did not feel able to consult the GP again herself as she had done so in the past without any result and this had created some ill-feeling between herself and the GP. I agreed to speak to the GP on her and her son's behalf.'

The health visitor had checked her assessment of the problem not only with the boy but also with his mother. She was clear about how anxious the boy was to overcome the problem and was aware that the full range of treatments had not been tried. It is apparent from the wording of this account that the health visitor was in sympathy with what the boy wanted and that she was prepared to represent his wants to the GP. The mother's support strengthened her advocacy. The fact that the family had already tried approaching the doctor but ill-feeling had strained their relationship meant that further empowerment was not likely to be acceptable. The health visitor therefore explicitly agreed a contract under which she would put the case to the GP. In further explanation, she gave some details about the options and risks that she had considered before going on to tackle the doctor:

> 'I did consider trying some methods of treatment of my own, but these would be minimal without GP consent and had been tried previously anyway. The last resort was to change GP but this seemed rather drastic. I risked failing to convince the GP to reconsider the treatment and also risked destroying my own relationship with both GP and parent should I fail. But when I spoke to the GP on behalf of the boy he was extremely helpful. He had not intended to appear unsympathetic to the boy or his mother, but felt that they had not stated their wants clearly enough. After discussion and because he felt that perhaps the boy's faith in him had taken a knock, he referred the boy to a paediatrician at the hospital for further investigations and a treatment programme. I consider this to be a successful outcome as both the boy and his mother respected the GP again, the boy would receive the treatment he needed and I remained on good terms with everyone.'

They do not always work out as well as that case, but part of the reason for the success was the accuracy of the health visitor's assessment and her clear understanding of the advocacy role. It also shows that conflict is not inevitable in advocacy. The agreement of a contract was made easier because the mother was supportive of her son. In some situations where family dynamics are complex, or where several people within a family have conflicting health care needs, advocates must make a clear decision about which family members they are representing.

An example of how to handle this type of situation was given by a district nurse who was called in to see an elderly patient. The man was being given diuretics as part of his treatment for heart failure but had become incontinent:

'The patient has recently moved to this area after the recent death of his wife and is in a very frail condition. He is being looked after by his son who has taken early retirement initially to look after and spend more time with his wife, who is just receiving a second course of radiotherapy treatment for a recurrence of cancer. I am particularly aware of the tremendous burden of support taken on by the son but realise that I cannot be an advocate for each person in the triangle at the same time. The father is very demanding and needs motivating. He is grieving heavily for his wife and for the change in his lifestyle. In recognising his daughter-in-law's problems, he feels a burden on everyone. The daughter-in-law is very depressed at her own illness and very concerned for her husband's problems in looking after both of them. The son/husband has divided loyalties, is exhausting himself trying to do everything, and has no time for his own grief. I have decided that since I was called in to see the father, my primary advocacy lies with him. If I can support him and let him express his feelings, it may help him to accept rest care or day care facilities to let the son and his wife spend time together on their own. But the father needs to know that I am really on his side or he will distrust my motives in suggesting these ideas. What I have also done, however, is liaise closely with the GP and the health visitor, and they are acting more as advocates for the husband and wife.'

This example shows how conflicts of interest can arise, even within a loving family. An advocate cannot represent two people whose wants are different, hence the need to be clear who is the primary client and at the same time to ensure that others affected also have helpers on their side. Another frequent complication occurs when patients are unable to express their wants, for example when very weak or overwhelmed with pain. Under these circumstances helpers may make common sense assumptions about what patients would want if only they were able to speak for themselves. However, it is good practice to discuss these assumptions with others before proceeding. This 'test by publicity' is one of the few ways of protecting silent patients from misdirected advocacy. An example concerns a patient with a nose bleed which had continued intermittently for 24 hours:

'The locum doctor repacked the nose twice more with no improvement. The patient was getting distressed and there was a great deal of blood loss including large clots. He was also vomiting stale blood. I had a word with the doctor concerned and suggested we call in the consultant, but he refused saying there wasn't a problem and he would come back in another hour and repack if there was no improvement. I contacted the corporate nurse for the hospital and told her about the situation. I said I felt I couldn't let things carry on but the doctor was not prepared to take advice. I said that I wanted to ring the consultant and asked her if she agreed. She said that if I was sure of my facts then she would support me. So I decided to plead the cause and went over the head of the doctor by ringing the consultant. I explained the situation, he came in, examined the patient and then took him to theatre and inserted a post-nasal pack that stopped the bleeding.'

In part the nurse's action in consulting the corporate nurse was a sensible measure to reduce the risk to her from a complaint by the locum doctor. But it also provided a test by publicity, enabling her to check her own view of the situation with that of a colleague who was willing to consider matters on behalf of a patient in no position to speak up for himself.

Planning

Moving from negotiating a contract to preparing to act as an advocate, the first element in planning is the acquisition of information. The amount of information needed will vary greatly from one situation to another. In some cases the advocate will already know enough about the technical details of the illness or treatment to be able to argue the case with no further research. However, if resistance is expected, supplementary information or revision of key facts may be required. In practice, the collection of up to date information frequently has less to do with constructing an argument than with establishing the credibility of the advocate in the eyes of those in authority. As well as researching technical details, advocates also need to be sure that they have sufficient information about their clients' personal circumstances and individual wants in order to represent them effectively. There are direct similarities here with the role of the legal advocate who has to master a brief in order to represent a client in the courts. Mastery of the brief will include information about what has happened to lead up to the case, technical details about the law and how it applies to this particular situation, and information about the client as a person so that the human side of the problem can be included in the argument.

An example which emphasises the information required to prepare a case was given by a staff nurse working in the community whose patient had some pressure sores which had taken 18 months to heal up in a specialist unit. The patient had now been discharged home but was recommended not to sit on a normal toilet seat in case his fragile skin suffered damage. Therefore he was having to manage at home with suppositories and to have his bowels open on the bed, which he felt was very undignified:

'I asked the specialist unit if they could recommend a special seat to fit over his toilet so he could have his bowels open normally. They recommended a very expensive seat. The patient did not have much money and could not afford to buy it. I asked my district nurse how we could obtain the seat and she suggested I wrote to the senior nurse requesting the purchase of this equipment by the Trust for which I worked. I discussed obtaining the seat with the patient and he approved of my writing the letter. He was disabled and could not write himself. I checked the details of the seat and price with the manufacturer, then wrote a letter explaining details of the equipment and where it was obtainable from. I also put the case based on the psychological importance for this patient of being able to have his bowels open normally. Finally I explained why this equipment was necessary in view of the patient's (expensive) past medical history. The letter was successful and we obtained the seat.'

Another element in preparation is to decide on the tactics which will be employed. The word tactics is deliberately chosen, with its connotations of short term planning, manipulation of a situation and recognition of the potential for conflict. Because advocacy is about power, a useful way of beginning to consider tactics is through an analysis of the nature of power. Charles Handy (1985) has put forward a typology which begins by differentiating between positive power and negative power. Positive power is the ability to create change and negative power is the ability to block it. Negative power is latent and does not operate all the time. Patients possess a great deal of negative power but do not always know how to use it, so some empowering approaches are designed to help patients to say no and to be heard when doing so. In contrast, an external advocate is usually trying to exercise positive power in order to plead for a change in the patient's situation. The third party in the relationship will by definition also hold a certain amount of power, which may be positive or negative or both. When planning tactics, advocates need to compare their own sources of power with those of the third party involved and this is made easier by considering Handy's (1985) list of five different types of power:

(1) Physical
(2) Resource
(3) Position
(4) Expert
(5) Personal.

Physical power

This is the power of physical force or coercion. It is not generally legitimate in our society to use physical power, but sometimes an advocate may meet resistance based on the threat of it. Physical power also includes the use of verbal aggression or a loud and hectoring tone to overcome opposition. I am not suggesting that this is a good way for an advocate to behave, but it may be important to have a response prepared in case a third party resorts to these tactics.

Resource power

This is the possession of valued resources which provide a useful basis for influencing others. It is the power to reward or to withhold rewards. In health care it will include command over a budget with sums available for staffing or non-pay resources. At a simpler level it may be the power to allow another person to use a telephone or a separate room. Advocacy will sometimes lead to a negotiation where each party controls resources which the other desires, leading to an 'if you will do this then I will agree to do that' type of bargain.

Position power

This is closely linked to resource power. Position power comes as a result of the roles which individuals hold within an organisation and its extent and legitimacy are conferred by the organisation, or in some cases by society as a whole. Position power frequently conveys control over resources, but in addition gives control over invisible assets such as the right of access to particular individuals or groups, the right to hold or withhold information, and the right to decide how things will be done. One of the problems for professionals who undertake health care advocacy within their own organisations is that their position power is likely to be weaker than that of the third party with whom they are dealing. However, independent advocates are by definition external or separate from the organisation where they practise their advocacy and so their position power is also limited, although they may hold some power if the health care organisation recognises the advocacy organisation as a truly legitimate part of the system.

Expert power

This is the power that derives from expertise or established specialist experience. Charles Handy makes the point that expert power is comparative – even a small differential in expertise can give one great power over others, provided that expertise happens to be in demand. Another point emphasised by Handy is that expertise only translates into expert power if others recognise and respect it. This is a frequent problem for non-medical staff who may have considerable expertise in specialist areas, but if this is not recognised by the doctors their expert power is very limited. In health care, with its many specialties and formal respect for scientific knowledge, expert power that can be established beyond doubt is particularly effective as a basis for advocacy.

Personal power

This is the power of personality or charisma. It is like a magical addition to expert or position power. Charles Handy cautions that many people believe they hold personal power until they lose their position in the organisation and discover that no one pays attention to their views any more. However, it is possible to build personal power on a foundation of trust which is slowly extended over a period of time. This is why some individuals are particularly powerful advocates with certain other individuals within an organisation.

Power tactics

A health visitor gave an example of the conscious use of power in everyday advocacy when she described the problems of a mother living in a high rise tower block with two very active sons:

'One son had been diagnosed as hyperactive and the younger son was in the process of being diagnosed. The husband was in the RAF and had approached the Families Officer for a change of house, but he had been refused. Because of this he was extremely reluctant to try again in case it was put down on his official record and damaged his career prospects. At the same time mum was being treated for depression and I was visiting to give the family support.

I approached the doctor who was assessing the boys and he gave me a written statement confirming he thought a move would benefit the children. I then made an appointment to see the Families Officer. My husband is in the RAF so I understand the way the service works. I made a point when I went into the office to "Sir" the officer at every opportunity, along the lines of, "Thank you sir for agreeing to this appointment. May I say, sir, that I understand the pressures and constraints there are on you . . ." etc. Then when I saw this was having an effect I began deliberately using plenty of medical terminology about the condition of the children and family in order to impress him, as well as bringing out the supporting letter from the specialist doctor. In fact he very quickly conceded the need for a move and said that he had a place since someone was just in the process of transferring to another RAF base. The family were moved within ten days.'

The health visitor had no position power or resources with which to bargain, since she was putting a case to a member of a different organisation. In this case she went out of her way to show that she recognised the important position of the Families Officer by 'sirring' him as much as possible. This flattered his dignity and put him in a mood to listen. The health visitor then established her claim to expert power in health care. Her deliberate use of medical jargon was designed to impress and the letter from the specialist merely confirmed her own expertise. In this case the expert power was not challenged by the third party because it was outside his own area of expertise, but he felt secure because of the respect shown to his rank and position. The manipulative elements in this interaction are immediately apparent. How far to go down this line must be a matter for individual judgement.

This issue of how far to go in using manipulation as a tactic in advocacy is made even more complicated by male-female dynamics. A nurse working in intensive care described a conflict over the treatment of an 85 year old woman who had been provisionally diagnosed as having had a heart attack, although the signs and symptoms were not conclusive. A registrar had prescribed streptokinase, which is an important drug in limiting the damage caused by heart attacks but also has dangerous side effects that need careful monitoring. The nurse had worked in the unit for some time and believed the woman might be suffering from a chest infection which could be presenting as a heart attack. The patient already had low blood pressure and this nurse had seen other patients die when streptokinase was administered under these circumstances.

She directly challenged the registrar's prescription, saying that streptokinase can lower blood pressure even further. The doctor was annoyed at this and stood on his dignity, stating that low blood pressure is not a formal contraindication for use of this drug. The nurse immediately recognised that she was not going to get anywhere using this tack and deliberately softened her approach, saying how worried she was about the woman's breathing difficulties and wondered if the doctor would mind listening to the patient's chest to see if she was imagining things or not. This was a deliberate ploy, using a soothing tone to reduce conflict and designed to get the doctor to prescribe an antiobiotic while believing that he had thought of it himself. It worked. The doctor prescribed the antibiotic augmentin and the patient rapidly improved. The nurse explained that she adopted this subservient role quite deliberately in order to get what she wanted for the patient. She had doubts about the morality of it and whether it was right for someone in her profession to lower herself in this way and also resented the arrogance of the doctor in not recognising her expertise. In an ideal world this kind of manipulation would not be necessary, although one could also argue that advocacy itself would hardly be required if we all behaved rationally and reasonably all the time.

Presenting the client's case

Bad presentation can spoil a good case so it is important for advocates to master some of the basic rules. Drummond (1990) gave a useful list which applies well to advocacy:

- Clarity
- Simplicity
- Brevity
- Liveliness
- Integrity
- Quiet assertiveness.

Clarity is achieved by assuming no detailed prior knowledge of the case by the third party. Then follows the classic sequence of telling the person what you are going to tell them, telling them, and finally telling them what you told them. Simplicity means being as straightforward as possible and in a case that involves numbers or sums of money to cut out the irrelevant detail and simply present the bottom line figures. Brevity is necessary in the high pressure world of modern health care. In complex cases it is a good idea to practise what you are going to say beforehand and to watch your timing. Liveliness means capturing and retaining the attention of whoever is listening. Above all this means telling the case as a story and bringing in the human feelings of the person represented:

'Mrs X was really pleased after she plucked up courage to ring the housing department. She opened the letter next day in eager antici-pation. Imagine her shock and disappointment when she saw what it said . . .' etc.

Integrity is about being straight and honest with the third party. It is usually better to establish and maintain a reputation for integrity as an advocate and steadily build up your status, rather than to sacrifice everything in a desperate attempt to cut corners and win a single case. Quiet assertiveness means treating the listeners as responsible adults with an interest in natural justice. This is not entirely compatible with the manipulative tactics described earlier. A compromise may be to begin by using quiet assertiveness and only to adopt manipulative tactics when it becomes apparent that the third party is not behaving in an entirely rational or reasonable way. The following community example shows the value of the assertive approach:

'The patient was an elderly gentleman whom we were already visiting for a dressing to his left leg. When I visited he told me that the right one had also started to trouble him. He was also very chesty. His leg was inflamed, had broken down in a couple of places and was blistered and tender to touch. I enquired if he had contacted the doctor and he replied that he had the previous day regarding his bad chest, but the doctor had told him to send his son for some medication. I said, "Didn't you ask for a visit?" He said that the doctor never visited him and had told his son that if he wasn't happy he could change doctors. So I said, "Well why don't you? You're much nearer to the other surgery." He also said that when he went to visit the doctor it cost him £3:20 in taxi fares as they had no transport.

I agreed to contact his GP for him and I also urged him to consider changing his doctor in the future. I agreed to make contact because I did not want to initiate any treatment until his doctor had seen his leg. I knew that this GP could be very difficult as another colleague had recently had problems getting him to visit a patient and was told, "You nurses want more professional responsibility but are not prepared to take responsibility for your actions". I contacted the GP and was told he would leave some antibiotics out for the patient, but I said, "He needs a visit – please go". It was not right to prescribe tablets on my description of the patient's symptoms. The doctor visited the patient. Tablets were prescribed for the infection in his chest but he was also discovered to have a deep vein thrombosis in his right leg. The patient has now decided with the rest of the family to transfer to another surgery and I consider my intervention to have been successful.'

The basis of the nurse's persistent assertiveness was her certainty that her judgement was sound. She knew that the pain and inflammation in the right leg had to be taken seriously and she also understood that the GP's contract with the health authority required him to visit a patient on request. She was prepared for opposition from the doctor but insisted he saw the patient with an assertive turn of phrase that did not permit any further prevarication. Her assessment of the risks to the patient was surely accurate and she appears to have been prepared to face the doctor's displeasure with equanimity.

Summary of key points

- External advocacy is necessary when clients have either exhausted the avenues open to them or when they are in no fit state to plead their own case
- If an advocate agrees to take on a case it is good practice to negotiate a clear contract with the client
- The test of publicity means talking with colleagues, relatives or others about proposed advocacy; it is an important safeguard for silent clients
- Planning advocacy involves estimating the relative power of the various parties involved and working to strengthen one's own power or to weaken that of unreasonable third parties
- Manipulative tactics are certainly used in everyday advocacy – it is a matter for individual conscience how far to go in this direction
- Presentation of a case begins with quiet assertion of a clear message.

Chapter 8
Reducing the Risks

It should be clear by now that advocacy can be a risky business for all concerned. It occurs in situations where emotions tend to be running high and it may involve a power struggle in which a weaker party is trying to be assertive in relation to a stronger party. There are risks to patients, who may lose heart if their attempts to speak up for themselves are not successful, or who may lose confidence in all the professionals involved if some do not seem to be listening. There are also risks to the third parties involved when clumsy attempts to assert patients' rights may lead to loss of temper and consequent misjudgements, particularly when advocacy is interpreted as a personal attack on an individual. However, this chapter places its focus firmly on the risks to the helpers or advocates, whether health care professionals or independent advocates. The justification for this emphasis is that these are the people who initiate advocacy or promote empowerment and therefore they are the ones who have most control over events and are in the best position to reduce the risks to all parties.

Forecasting the risks

As an advocate or helper it is very easy to get caught up in emotional outrage at the ways in which patients are treated or mistreated. It is this sense of outrage that gives courage and purpose to advocacy. However, if the heart is allowed to overrule the head, the risks to all parties increase as conflict for its own sake becomes more likely. In practical terms, effective advocates are able to control their moral outrage and adopt assertive, but not aggressive, approaches, even in the most difficult situations. An important safeguard is to try to forecast the possible risks *before* deciding whether or not to pursue a case. This is the same process that legal teams go through in deciding whether to pursue a case through the courts, agree to an out of court settlement, or abandon the case entirely. This legal analogy is quite close to the reality of health care advocacy. The 'out of court settlement' is similar to a direct approach to the third party involved where, as a result of negotiation, an agreement acceptable to everyone involved is arrived at. 'Going to court' in terms of health care advocacy means going over the head of the third party to try to get a judgement from someone more senior and more powerful. The highest court is the court of publicity invoked by whistleblowers. 'Abandoning a case' is sometimes just as necessary in health care as in law. It does not mean abandoning the patient, but it does involve a recognition that at that particular moment the patient's wants cannot be met in the way the patient would like. Barristers as professionals do not expect to succeed in every case. It is the same for advocates involved in health care: some cases will be won and some will be lost. It is the reality of everyday advocacy. Accurate forecasting of risk at an early stage is therefore essential and should include the following:

- The nature of the issue
- The differences between advocacy for individuals and for groups
- The different contractual positions of professional and independent advocates
- The type of advocacy proposed.

Forecasting begins by examining the issues in question. Chapter 2 reviewed several cases including that of Graham Pink, the charge nurse who complained about low staffing levels at night on an elderly care ward. According to Mihill (1991) Mr Pink began by going through his line management and even succeeded in getting the person in charge of the hospital to visit the ward one night. It appears that he initially believed the problem was one of communication, reasoning that the senior people in the hospital did not realise that staffing levels were very low in relation to patient dependency. If this information could be communicated effectively to them – for example if they could see what was happening with their own eyes – they would be bound to agree to increase staffing. As we know, it did not work out like that. The senior managers either disagreed with Mr Pink's judgement of staffing levels or were constrained by other priorities so they could not accede to what was wanted. In other words, the situation was not a communication problem but a problem of substance with strongly held views on both sides. Problems of substance entail greater risk than simple communication problems, since by definition they involve conflicting views.

In addition, Graham Pink was acting as an advocate for all the patients on the ward and all the people who could potentially be admitted to that ward in the future. Advocacy on behalf of a group of people almost always carries greater risks than advocacy on behalf of one or two individuals. The extent of the change that the group advocate is seeking is likely to be larger and will usually cost more money to implement than when acting for an individual. Also the extent of the implied criticism of people in authority is frequently greater, since they may see themselves as accused of prolonged failure to recognise a problem, the scale of which opens them to charges of negligence. The obvious form of defence is to argue that there is no problem at all and that the individual making all the fuss is a malicious troublemaker. Advocacy on behalf of groups may therefore be seen as a form of political action and this may be viewed as an illegitimate activity for an individual, particularly if that individual is an employee of the organisation which is being criticised. An independent advocate will carry fewer risks in this type of situation than a professional under contract. By signing a contract, one accepts a duty of loyalty towards one's employer which may be breached by vigorous advocacy, particularly where it involves going public through whistleblowing. In contrast the independent advocate is expected to speak up for clients and in many cases will not be an employee of the organisation being criticised and therefore will be less vulnerable to loss of job based on breach of contract.

Any estimate of risk must take into account the type of helping approach proposed. As a general rule, empowerment approaches carry less risk, at least to the helper, than external advocacy. In external advocacy the helpers make themselves visible to those in power through the very act of speaking up on behalf of someone else. They are also vulnerable if their assessment of clients' wants is inaccurate or if clients change their minds. In contrast, empowerment approaches place clients in the forefront, with helpers in a supporting role. The risks arising from clients changing their minds are also virtually eliminated in empowerment since they become the sole responsibility of the clients themselves. A further consideration, which applies particularly to external advocacy, is how far the advocate is prepared to take the case. Advocacy that involves going through the formal channels within an organisation is less risky than jumping levels in the hierarchy and appealing over the head of the third party. The greatest risks arise from going outside the organisation to pursue the case, particularly in whistleblowing which involves going to the press or other media.

The decision whether or not to pursue a particular case and, if so, how best and how far to pursue it, remains a matter for individual conscience. However it is certainly good practice to choose one of the lower risk options when these are available and offer a reasonable chance of success. In particular, the choice of empowerment over external advocacy reduces the risk to all parties. Equally, it is important to recognise right from the start that high risk external advocacy may affect other people who are close to us in our own lives. Family, friends and colleagues may become caught up in the stress of events, or may be affected emotionally, economically or socially by the fall-out. This does not mean that high risk approaches should never be used, but it does suggest prior consultation with family or friends.

Different aspects of risk and how to reduce them

Analysis of the literature suggests that risks may be divided into three aspects:

(1) Effects on self-esteem
(2) Effects on future working relationships
(3) Effects of being labelled a troublemaker.

Self-esteem

Failure as a helper is an obvious source of harmful effects, such as the feeling that one has let the client down, perhaps having promised a particular outcome or having allowed oneself to be seen as a more powerful protector than was in fact the case. An example given in interview by a theatre nurse clarifies the issues involved:

'The surgeon was annoyed with the patient and it wasn't the patient's fault. It was a dental operation under local anaesthetic and the patient was in pain, she was frightened. And I don't think the surgeon should have carried on. It was only a short procedure, a removal of a tooth or a couple of teeth. But she was frightened. And we stopped once and gave her some more analgesia, but she still complained of pain. The surgeon carried on regardless. He went quite quickly, but it was obviously a bad experience for her ... I was trying to go between the patient and the surgeon, trying to reassure the patient saying, "It's only a little bit more", or something like that. It puts you in a difficult position because you can't say, "Stop, you should stop this". You can suggest but you can't insist ... And I don't think the patient felt able to say to him "Stop". which would be quite within her rights ... I asked him to stop once, because she was obviously feeling pain. But time was getting on and he wanted to get finished. He did stop once but then went on ... I suggested he stopped again, saying she had had enough. But he said he would just finish it off quickly, which he did. I felt angry and sorry for the patient. It sticks in my mind even though it was a year ago.'

The nurse was visibly still upset by the situation when she recounted it, despite the passage of time. She had tried to speak up on behalf of the patient, but felt in the end that she had in some way failed. Accepting the realities of power in the situation, what can be done to reduce the advocate's loss of self-esteem? A first step is to review significant events like this with another person, such as a clinical supervisor or a close and trusted friend. The other person can provide a sounding board as the nurse questions whether there was anything more that could be done. In this situation the nurse tried intervening twice. Her statement that she could not insist on the surgeon stopping the operation is accurate. Ultimately this comes down to the patient. If the patient was not pre-pared to indicate unequivocally that she wanted the operation to be stopped, the nurse could do no more than she did. There may be implications for the future. Perhaps the nurse could have helped herself by explaining her views to the surgeon afterwards. If the patient wished later to complain about her treatment an empowering approach to help her understand the complaints procedure could have been adopted. But in the matter in question, the nurse needed someone else to tell her that she had done all that could reasonably be expected of her in the situation and that she is allowed to let herself off the hook.

While empowerment for self-advocacy may not be a realistic option in the middle of an operation, it is certainly consciously adopted by many helpers when they believe that the risk of harm to their credibility from failed advocacy is too great. A school nurse described this quite explicitly when working with the mother of a child who had been excluded from two schools because of aggressive behaviour:

'I discussed the problem with mother and child. The mother wanted me to offer help to the child and then go to the school and speak up to get him reinstated. Instead I suggested that the mother should go to her GP and seek help from the child guidance service. I felt unable to deal with this myself and thought that someone who specialised in child behaviour problems could be of more help. I felt also that the child's chances of being reinstated in school would be increased if help was being sought from a specialist. I felt the risk to me, if I took the case on with the school and failed, was my credibility with the family. I also felt very strongly that I would serve a greater purpose by preserving my relationship with the family and keeping open the link between home and school. The mother could be a very volatile lady. The mother did go to the GP, and the child guidance service has agreed to regular appointments for mother and child to work on behaviour strategies. This outcome is successful in that the child has been seen quickly and moves have been made to allow him back into school, although I am unsure of how cooperative the parent will continue to be.'

Essentially the school nurse was trying to shape the mother's expectations of her to make them more realistic. She did not fall into the trap of promising successful advocacy when it could not be delivered. Even though she may have lost some credibility in the first instance, she preserved her longer term relationship with the family and her own self esteem by deliberately choosing empowerment over advocacy in this situation.

Future working relationships

Giving health care is a team enterprise with each individual depending on others for support, advice and help. Already from the examples in this book we have seen the way that some powerful individuals misinterpret and resent the challenge from an advocate. Some people bear grudges and use patients as pawns in a power game to seek revenge. This can affect independent advocates just as much as professionals, since the third party may deny the independent advocate future access to patients or necessary information about their condition. Grudges most frequently arise from advocacy which involves going over the head of the third party, but they can also be associated with empowerment where the third party believes that information should not have been given to the patient by the helper.

For every helper, some working relationships will be more important than others. It is vital to anticipate events and calculate whether you can afford to damage your relationship with the particular third party involved. Generally speaking, assertive approaches are less likely to cause long term relationship problems than either aggressive or manipulative techniques. If it is possible to keep calm and simply repeat the message until the resistance is worn down (the 'broken record' technique described by Dickson 1982), the third party may end up feeling exasperated rather than personally attacked. This method works well in situations where the problem is more one of communication than of substance. In contrast, manipulative approaches may give short-term successes but they tend to store up problems for the future. Individuals are likely to feel aggrieved if advocates appeal over their heads to more senior people in the organisation without being assertive enough to explain the situation directly to them in the first place.

A useful way of reducing the risk of future relationships is to talk-up one's advocacy role before using it. For example, the job descriptions of some health care professionals now include acting as the patient's advocate. This is helpful because it gives staff official sanction to take on advocacy and can form a defence in the event of complaints. It is even more useful if other professionals in positions of authority have been reminded that advocacy is part of the role. This means stating it clearly in case conferences and other discussions: 'As you know, being an advocate for patients is part of my job description, so I am sure you will appreciate why I want to bring this particular problem to your attention'. In the same way, it is important to address controversial issues over treatment policies, truth telling and the authority of different members of the team at times when everyone is calm and before difficult situations have to be dealt with. One Macmillan nurse that I interviewed appeared to be an especially strong empowerer of patients with maximum discretion to give information, even when it was bad news. When I questioned the nurse about this, it became apparent that the difficult issues had been carefully addressed within the team well in advance:

'I discussed the policy on disclosure with the medical staff when I first started this job. I would never deliberately go out of my way to give people information about diagnosis, but I would if I felt it right; if I felt they were definitely asking for information and it was information which I had, then I would give them that. It is a general policy agreed right throughout the hospital fortunately. It's been discussed with management and it's backed up by the UKCC, that nobody, but nobody, can force us to lie. I had one case recently where a relative was adamant and put it in writing, almost a legal type of thing, that he didn't want any information about diagnosis given to the patient. He was seen by me and a member of the medical staff to explain that we basically couldn't hold to that. Legally the contract is between the doctor, other professionals, and the patient. But it had to be also explained to him in the same breath that we heard what he said. And we would only give information if the patient almost dragged it out of us, and if the patient asked about cancer we would rebound the question on him. And we in a sense gave the relative some scenarios about how we would handle it. And the other thing that reassured the relative is if we did give any information we would keep the relatives informed of what had been asked and what we had said.'

So here was an area where potential problems had been worked through well in advance. Roles were clear and accepted and could be sustained even in the face of a legalistic challenge from a relative. Contrast this with a situation in a different hospital where a patient was suffering from terminal cancer:

'All the time we could see that he was deteriorating. We kept getting the feeling that he wanted to know what was happening but the consultant in particular was very evasive. Then a friend of the patient who was a GP came in to see him. And he asked him outright, "Am I going to die, am I going to get any better?" And the GP told him straight, "No you're not going to get any better." I had discussed this possibility with the GP earlier as I felt that the consultant was wrong in some respects. Everyone on the ward had grown attached to the patient and we were finding it difficult that there was this sort of barrier, "Do we say or do we not?". And it's almost like everybody was role acting. I was going off duty for the weekend so I let this member of staff know that the patient knew his prognosis. Unfortunately this member of staff didn't pass it on to the others. So consequently at the weekend the patient needed to talk but the staff carried on being evasive. I wasn't able to recapture the relationship, I think it shattered a lot of trust. By the time I'd come back from the weekend the patient had already rapidly begun to deteriorate.'

The nurses in this situation accepted the consultant's right to control disclosure of information, even though they disagreed with it. Instead of assertively discussing this with the consultant, a GP was used as a safe vehicle for disclosing the information and technically empowering the patient with minimal risk of backlash from the consultant onto the staff. However, this in itself revealed to the patient that the whole team had been withholding information and so must have damaged his trust in them. Then the failure to communicate what the patient knew to the rest of the team did further harm and deprived him of the close relationships that he needed in his final few days. The root of the problem was a lack of assertiveness on the part of all the professionals in the hospital team, leading to manipulative methods of tackling problems and disastrous consequences for at least one patient.

Being labelled a troublemaker

This is the most serious risk for any advocate. It is the one that threatens future job security and current or future relationships. It is what happened to Graham Pink (Mihill 1991) and to Jolene Tuma (Kohnke 1982, pp. 23–24). It occurs when groups of senior people within an organisation come to regard an individual as a problem to be eliminated, rather than a voice to be heard. If the matter is one of substance and the advocate is prepared to go as far as whistleblowing, then the trouble-maker label is almost certain to be applied. So what can be done? The first line of defence is to seek safety in numbers. If one person peeks over the parapet that person can be shot down, but if a large number of people arise to be counted, they cannot be picked off so easily. This means seeking support from colleagues and agreeing to support one another. Very often this is best achieved through a trades union or professional organisation. In one NHS Trust a health visitor campaigned with a group of parents for improvements to a block of flats which were damp and were causing health problems to the children. A national newspaper got to hear of the story and rang the health visitor for a comment. Fortunately she had her wits about her and said she would ring them back. In the meantime she contacted her professional organisation where she was advised to speak to the reporter as someone representing the views of the association, rather than as an employee of an NHS Trust. This made her relatively safe from accusations of disloyalty to her employer, so she could express herself more freely and in more political terms than would otherwise have been wise.

Additional help in high pressure situations is available from the charity Public Concern at Work. Their 1997 review of activities contains two patient-care case studies which highlight the type of legal advice and practical support they can offer. The first involved the deputy matron of a nursing home who suspected that the person who ran the home was sexually abusing vulnerable residents. The charity was able to advise her about the strength of evidence that would be required in order to go public by contacting the police and presenting them with enough material to give them a reasonable chance of pursuing a criminal charge. The deputy matron did what she could to protect the residents. But when an incident occurred despite her vigilance, she collected a specimen that was confirmed as semen when tested by a forensic laboratory, paid for by the charity. She was then able to go to the police with some confidence and the evidence was sufficient to convict the guilty party while protecting the reputation and employment of the deputy matron.

The second case study concerned a day care assistant at a private rest home who found evidence that a colleague was mistreating residents. The owner of the home said he would sort the matter out but nothing changed. The assistant mentioned the situation to a local authority inspector visiting the home and this led to a referral to the police. However, the day care assistant was suspended as well as the colleague accused of mistreating the patients. Two weeks later the assistant got a letter from the owner telling her to return to work but also saying she was to receive a written warning because she had broken her contract of confidentiality and damaged the reputation of the home. It was at this point that she contacted Public Concern at Work. Support was given over the telephone. It was clear that the assistant liked working in the home and did not wish to push the situation into open conflict by asserting her legal rights or having the charity write a lawyer's letter to the owner. Instead they drafted a letter for the assistant to send which apologised for any inconvenience, explained the reasons for her actions and pointed out that she had not herself called in the police. The outcome was that the written warning was withdrawn and the assistant was welcomed back to work, thus defusing the situation in the way that she wanted.

Public Concern at Work is campaigning to persuade more employers in both public and private sectors to create policies on whistleblowing, recognising that front line employees are usually the first to recognise possible misconduct and therefore need the encouragement and support of a formal policy to create an atmosphere of openness within the organisation. In dealing with concerns they urge all parties to recognise that there are two sides to every story, that employees may have legitimate concerns about their own safety or career, that victimising employees is a disciplinary offence as are malicious counter-accusations, and that senior managers should commit themselves to report back to employees concerned on the outcome of any investigations.

Summary of key points

- The basis of reducing risk in advocacy is to forecast potential risks before taking action and to apply safeguards to stop the most serious risks becoming a reality
- Clarity and realism about patients' rights provide a sound basis for empowerment or external advocacy
- Empowerment for self-advocacy is preferable to external advocacy since it is less risky for the advocate and promotes independence in the patient
- It is protective to establish advocacy formally as part of your role: for example through job descriptions, whistleblowing policies and talking-up the role
- It is valuable to enlist advice and support early-on from independent advocates, trades unions, professional organisations, charity bodies such as Public Concern at Work and trusted colleagues
- An assertive approach (rather than a manipulative one) tends to minimise damage to future relationships
- Above all, use your moral outrage, but don't let it use you.

Chapter 9
Advocacy Schemes for People with Special Needs

Many independent advocacy schemes have started by working in partnership with individuals with special advocacy needs, including for example those whose problems arise from learning disabilities, mental illness, or the effects of the ageing process. In an ideal world no one would have special advocacy needs because our society as a whole would listen and respond to all its members. The reality is that we are all limited in our responses by ignorance, prejudice and preconception. Special needs require special resources in a democratic society, including good quality independent advocacy support. This chapter does not attempt to provide an all-inclusive directory of special advocacy schemes, but instead tries to illustrate the nature of this type of advocacy, drawing on the experience of schemes from three areas:

- People with learning disabilities
- Older people
- People from ethnic minority backgrounds.

Learning disabilities

One of the first advocacy schemes for people with learning disabilities was established in the USA by Wolf Wolfensberger in the mid 1960s (Wertheimer 1993). Wolfensberger was challenged at a conference by the parents of children with learning disabilities. These parents recognised their own role as advocates for their children, but they were desperately anxious about who would speak up for the children when they as the parents were no longer alive. The basic principles behind Wolfensberger's scheme were to promote the right to services based on individual needs, with protection from abuse and unnecessary restriction of rights. Many schemes in the UK have been driven by parents with similar concerns and have built on the same pioneering principles.

Another spur to action in this area has been an awareness that the institutions set up to support and care for individuals with learning disabilities sometimes fail to live up to their own high ideals. This is a particular problem when financial constraints lead those in authority to create plans for the future based on assumptions about the needs of groups, rather than the wants of individuals. A case study (Booth 1991) illustrates the vulnerability of individuals with learning disabilities to changes in the way services are organised.

> Henry O'Brien was first placed in an institution at the age of 15 and was subsequently moved 13 times. In the early 1980s he lived in a house in the grounds of an old hospital for the mentally handicapped, which offered greater independence to its residents than the wards of the main hospital. A shift in consultants' responsibilities led to him being moved back to the main hospital, where his condition began to deteriorate. His mother strongly opposed the move, acting as an advocate on his behalf, but was unable to stop it. Despite this Mr O'Brien was put forward for relocation to a local authority hostel under a community care programme that would move him closer to his parents. However, a series of changes overwhelmed his ability to cope. Another resident who was his closest friend was moved away to a different hostel; the occupational therapist who had worked with him left to take up a job elsewhere; and his father became seriously ill, meaning that visits home were restricted because his mother was having difficulty coping. These events proved too much for Mr O'Brien. He ran away from the hospital and slept rough for two days. On his return he was deemed no longer suitable for the move to a hostel and instead remained in the old hospital, becoming withdrawn, disorientated and incontinent despite all the years of expensive health care.

The argument which Wendy Booth (1991) puts forward in describing Mr O'Brien's case is that no one seemed to understand the emotional and psychological strains which a series of planned and unplanned changes had placed upon him. The institutions and the people who controlled them seemed oblivious to his needs as an individual because they were thinking at an organisational level, trying to reduce the number of hospital wards and set up hostels for the 'better' patients. Booth argues that an independent or citizen advocacy programme could have made a real difference:

> 'During the process of change there were many opportunities when a citizen advocate could have talked through with Henry the events that were undermining his stability and could have helped him to assert some control over the situation. To begin with, an advocate should

have been allocated to Henry when it was decided to include his name in the community care programme, especially when it was noted that his parents were coping with problems of their own. At all times, Henry's thoughts on the move needed checking out. For instance, did he want to go to this particular hostel? Were there any friends he would especially like to live with? What were his worries? Did he feel ready to move or would he prefer a delay until the distress occasioned by his father's illness had eased? Henry's feelings about these matters were critical and needed communicating to those responsible for his transfer.' (Booth 1991)

An example of the type of service which Booth was demanding is the Advocacy Alliance which was launched in the UK in 1982. It began by using long term partnerships to befriend, protect and represent residents in two large hospitals for people with learning disabilities (Sang & O'Brien 1984) and was sponsored by five national organisations: MIND, MENCAP, the Spastics Society, the Leonard Cheshire Foundation and One-to-One (Wertheimer 1993). Some of the problems associated with independent advocacy were addressed in the initial negotiations with the hospitals, which established a code of practice. This dealt with relationships between advocates, residents and care staff, the right of access to the resident by the advocate, the issue of confidentiality and confirmation that the advocate would not take on work that could be seen as the role of a member of the hospital staff (Gates 1994). Recruitment was slow, as is frequently the case in independent advocacy schemes for people with disabilities. Volunteers were trained over a three-month period and partnered over that time with the most appropriate residents. Difficulties included the considerable time demands required to establish an advocacy partnership, where frequent visits by the advocate at regular and predictable intervals were important. It also took advocates some time to understand the way that long years of institutionalisation had affected the ability of residents to relate to other people and the volunteers needed support at times when their help was rejected by individual residents.

In response to some of these difficulties with independent advocacy schemes, a self-advocacy movement has gained ground in recent years. According to Bob Gates:

'In this type of advocacy the advocate, or facilitator, attempts to shift the focus of control from him/herself to the people with whom he/she is working ... In self-advocacy people are encouraged to speak up for themselves, thus bringing about an element of self-empowerment, that is, people speaking for themselves rather than having an advocate speak for them. There is a strong ideological belief that self-advocacy enables people to grow and develop from the experience of speaking up for themselves. Growth in this context refers to both the enhancement and development of self-confidence and self-esteem.' (Gates 1994, p.4)

To promote self-advocacy, some training is usually needed for group members and for their supporters. A delicate balance has to be struck between helping individuals to participate as they choose in the group and trainers presenting lessons learned from the experience of others. Dawson and Palmer (1991) challenge service providers to look at issues such as policy making, service running, information sharing and training, and then ask how service users can have a say in these areas, what evidence there is that their contributions are valued, and what helps and what hinders self-advocacy. From this analysis, practical objectives for empowering service users can be established and pursued.

The particular strength of the self-advocacy movement is that these schemes bring people together in groups. This means that individuals can to some extent compensate for the disabilities of others. Also by putting forward views as a group they can exert more power and influence than by speaking up as isolated individuals. Now there is a risk that self-advocacy groups will be used by health authorities or social services departments as token participants in mock consultation exercises where views are respected only when they agree with those of the professionals (Simons 1992). However, determined groups can achieve practical changes. Whittaker (1988 and 1990) quotes examples of self-advocacy groups changing the way outsiders label them, winning a pay rise, and gaining access to meeting facilities away from service settings as a clear statement of their growing independence.

Older people

One of the driving forces behind independent action has been the consumer movement, reflected in political initiatives such as The Patient's Charter (Department of Health 1992). With many political thinkers urging a reduction in the role of the state in the provision of health and social services, the idea that individuals can and should influence the services which they choose to use is far more widely accepted than ever before. However, Wertheimer (1993) noted that although older people have concerns similar to those of the rest of the population, they are far less likely to complain or to seek information or advice, quoting from a study of choice and participation among older people:

'Consumer choice, when it was exercised by elderly people, usually took the form of refusing services that were offered or discontinuing them if they were found to be unsatisfactory. The general picture painted was that any participation and choice of the elderly people in the community in the services they received was essentially passive or negative. There was absolutely no sign of an active consumer movement among the elderly people interviewed either. They kept their heads down and tried to keep out of trouble. Complaining . . . was the last resort and very feared by some in case they were "crossed off the list".' (Allen *et al.* 1992, p.312)

Wertheimer (1993) therefore argues that at a time when major policy changes are being made in health and social services using the language of choice and participation as a justification, the elderly are in fact 'reluctant consumers' and can easily become victims to the way our society sidelines them, referring to them as a 'rising tide' or as a 'burden'. While many older people are well able to speak up for themselves, as a group they are subject to a succession of major transitions which would test the resilience of even the most articulate and empowered. These transitions are caused by the series of losses which arise both from the physical ageing process and from the isolation that is a feature of a society where children move away from their parents, where the low rate of the state pension makes older people dependent on dwindling savings, and where fear of crime is a deep-seated worry. One way in which advocacy services could become more effective for this group of reluctant consumers would be to focus on the fixed transition points which affect many elderly people. Where these transition points involve contact with health care or social services, it could be argued that funding derived from precisely these sources should be used to establish independent advocacy services. Examples of these transition points, based around the ideas of Wertheimer (1993), are:

(1) At the point of decision about hospital admission with advocacy contact through GPs' surgeries.
(2) When treatment options are presented, particularly to people suffering from cancer and where the choice is between aggressive surgical or radiotherapy interventions and more palliative approaches. Independent advocacy in these areas could supplement the work already done by hard-pressed specialist professionals, such as Macmillan nurses.
(3) Discharge from hospital and possible moves into residential or nursing home care, with advocacy services jointly supported by health and social services to ensure an independent voice speaking

up for the wants of the individual in the discharge planning process and beyond.

Wertheimer (1993) quotes a case study of Grace, an elderly widow with no close family who had fallen and fractured her hip. As she recovered in hospital, the professionals urged discharge into nursing home care rather than back to her own home. Grace was convinced she could manage at home. The ward staff contacted a local advocacy service on behalf of Grace but she declined the offer of an advocate. In the end she was reluctantly discharged into nursing home accommodation. She became desperately unhappy, refusing to eat and saying she wanted to go home. At this point she asked for an advocate and a partnership was established. The advocate fought long and hard on Grace's behalf to overcome professional scepticism and allow Grace to be discharged home with a range of support services. It would have been very difficult for the professionals involved to overcome the conflict of interest and concerns over risk which arose from Grace's wishes. On her own she could never have voiced her wants sufficiently forcefully. But with an independent advocate her argument that she had a right to live where she chose was properly heard and she was able to return home and maintain her chosen lifestyle.

People from ethnic minority backgrounds

'I have been doing this job for four years, and I would like to talk about my experiences. At first we had difficulty in getting people to accept that we weren't just interpreters. They kept asking us about our qualifications. We felt that we could speak for and help women of our communities through our own experiences. What we do is offer help and support in the clinics. We visit wards, run groups in hospitals and health centres and visit women at home.'

This is the voice of Zohra Ali Zubair, one of the workers employed on the Multi-Ethnic Women's Health Project in Hackney in the 1980s (Cornwell & Gordon 1984, p1). The project was funded by Inner City Partnership monies to provide a health advocacy and health advisory service for non-English speaking women in Hackney during pregnancy, childbirth and immediately afterwards. It was administered by the local Community Health Council and has provided a model from which many later schemes have developed. It aimed to improve access to health care, promote choice and informed decision-making, advise the health authority on policy and practice with regard to the needs of non-English speaking women and to help health care professionals improve their service to this high-risk group. The advocates were women from the relevant communities, chosen for commitment and experience rather than formal qualifications (Cornwell & Gordon 1984). The five workers, all part-time, comprised Turkish, Urdu, Gujurati and Bengali speakers.

Research by Waterson (1993) has shown that even after the Patient's Charter it still takes a great deal of patience and persistence to get information about maternity services from the service providers, even when the questioner is extremely persistent and has a strong health care background. How much more difficult therefore must it be for individuals whose culture and language is different from that of the service providers and where the fact of not speaking English exacerbates all the usual problems of feeling powerless in dealings with the professionals?

The Hackney project was definitely not an interpreting service therefore. The role of an interpreter is to find out from patients the answers to questions from the professionals and to tell the patients what the staff are going to do. The advocate's role is almost the exact opposite. It is to relay patients' questions and wants to the staff and to report back their answers:

> 'Nothing changes if there is just interpreting, it is a one-way process. We would merely have transmitted the hospital's wishes and instructions to the patient. We want much more than that. We want to defend and stand with the woman, make the woman's wishes known also to the hospital so that it is a real two-way process, not just in understanding language but in changing what goes on in hospital if it is unacceptable to our women.' (Shameem Habibullah quoted in Cornwell & Gordon 1984, p.18)

The project aimed not only to speak up for individuals but also to influence policy by getting the people in power to face up to the issue of racism in the treatment of patients from ethnic minorities. Examples which came to light included male students being brought in to see patients who have specifically asked to be seen only by a female doctor, midwives making up their own (English) names for the babies of non-English speaking women, and a hospital which claimed to provide vegetarian meals but in fact continued to use meat fats to cook the food. The project naturally aroused controversy and the presence of the advocates produced tensions with hospital staff, for example over the confidentiality of patients' notes. They were also met with accusations of stirring up racism where previously it had not existed. The advocates needed support from senior members of the hospital staff to be able to continue their work, while being accountable only to the project steering group within the Community Health Council.

> 'For the staff, there has been discomfort and distress at having their attitudes and work practices questioned by the Project workers as well as the initial fears among some that their jobs were under threat. The tension is less now partly because it has become clear that their areas of work do not overlap, but also because senior nurses spend time explaining the project and how it works to new members of staff. A minority of staff, notably among clerical and paramedical workers, continue to resent the workers.' (Cornwell & Gordon 1984, p.23)

Some statistical evidence for the effectiveness of the Hackney scheme was found in a retrospective study of 1000 non-English speaking women (Parsons & Day 1992). The study compared women who were accompanied by an advocate when delivering at the Mothers' Hospital in Hackney in 1986 with a reference group who had delivered without an advocate at Whipps Cross Hospital in 1979. The study found significant difference between the two groups, particularly a lower frequency of Caesarean section in Hackney. The authors acknowledged the limitations of the research, particularly the time difference between the two groups studied, but concluded that health advocacy may help to address some of the adverse obstetric outcomes observed in ethnic minority groups.

Conclusion

The projects described in this chapter highlight the strengths and weaknesses of independent advocacy schemes. It would be very difficult for the professionals within the health service to avoid conflicts of interest in advocating on behalf of specific groups of disadvantaged people, particularly where the wants of these groups have significant resource implications for the service providers. Advocacy on behalf of groups also has political undertones and is therefore an area where health care professionals are at risk. However, this is not to say that all is plain sailing for independent advocacy schemes. The search for stable funding is a constant worry. Even where social services or health authorities support such schemes, there is a fine balance between being effective and being independent which represents a continuing challenge to the long term future of independent advocacy schemes.

Summary of key points

- Independent advocacy schemes need careful planning and good liaison at senior levels with health care managers in order to gain and maintain access in the face of inevitable tensions with the professionals on the ground
- Selection of advocates is difficult, particularly where longer term partnership relationships are sought with groups of patients who may be reluctant users of advocacy services
- Considerable training is required to help the advocates balance their strong emotional commitment to their partners against the realities of power which mean they have to work with the system to some extent in order to maintain access and avoid rejection
- Despite all the difficulties, highly effective schemes have shown the way forward in improving services for people with learning disabilities, elderly people and mothers whose first language is not English.

Chapter 10
The Role of Patients' Relatives

A much-neglected aspect of advocacy is the role of patients' relatives. This chapter gives a brief introduction to advocacy as it affects relatives but does not pretend to provide a comprehensive treatment of this under-researched area. It looks at occasions when professionals feel they have to act as advocates against the wishes of relatives and also at occasions when relatives feel a need to advocate against professionals and on behalf of their loved ones. It is self evident that advocacy issues for relatives are approached from a viewpoint which is emotionally very different from that of the professionals and from that of independent advocates. The situations also vary according to whether the relatives are caring for the patient in the community or whether they are visitors to a hospital or other institution where the patient is being looked after by others. Another way of considering the involvement of relatives is to examine the differences between situations where patients are able to ask family members to act as advocates and those situations where the relatives assume the role without consulting the patient.

Care in the Community

Vast numbers of people, predominantly women, give their time to caring for sick or disabled family members in the community. They range from parents looking after their children all the way through to children caring for elderly parents, together with all the other permutations of family members and different types of involvement. Viewed from an advocacy perspective potential conflict most frequently occurs when a health care professional believes the care given by the relative is not meeting the patient's needs. In these circumstances, professionals are likely to consider taking up advocacy on behalf of the patient and against the relative. An example from a district nurse helps to clarify this:

'My patient was an elderly lady who had previously had a stroke and also suffered from a non-Hodgkin's lymphoma. The patient was being looked after by her husband and I began to suspect that he was abusing her. I noticed that she had bruises on her arms and one day when I visited I found her sitting on a commode, wet, with her husband refusing to help her or move her because she had wet herself before reaching the commode. Later I asked the patient on her own what the situation was and she admitted that her husband sometimes hit her, but she did not want me to do anything about it. She was very vulnerable. The husband defiantly admitted what was happening but said their marriage was none of my business. I discussed the problem with him and said it couldn't carry on. I reported the situation to the GP and contacted the day unit which the woman attended twice weekly. A social worker was contacted and also the police family support unit for advice. At a case conference we increased the respite and home care given to the patient and got her to attend the day unit three times a week. We made the husband aware that we were keeping an eye on him and were not intimidated physically by him.'

The district nurse was explicitly critical of the husband's care of his wife and directly challenged him about it. She sought a mandate from the patient to allow her to act as her advocate, but was given only partial support for this. We do not know the husband's point of view, whether he was at the end of his tether caring for his wife or whether he was simply malicious. The division of power in this situation was complex. The patient and her husband were in their own home, so the district nurse was a visitor who lacked position power. She did possess expert power and also a degree of personal power in being confident in asserting herself and confronting the husband. However, her mandate for advocacy was weakened by the woman's unwillingness to support further action. The husband evidently had physical power and also position power arising from control over access to the home. The basis for his personal power was his wife's willingness to continue to put up with the situation.

From an ethical perspective, the issue turns on how autonomous the woman continued to be. If she retained rational decision-making powers and trusted the professionals to protect her, then her refusal to support stronger action against her husband signified implicit consent to the status quo. On the other hand, if she was regarded as insufficiently autonomous to make a rational decision, the various authorities would have had greater freedom to protect her from harm, acting in a beneficent way. In the event, the district nurse ultimately felt she had to respect the patient's autonomy, while trying to convince the husband that she was prepared to take more drastic action to protect the patient if he did not mend his ways. An extension of this situation occurs in child protection cases where the moral imperative of beneficence is strengthened by legislation empowering the professionals to override the wishes of parents if it appears that child abuse is occurring in the home.

The situation discussed so far is one where outside professionals are explicitly critical of care provided by family members and seek to act as advocates to promote the best interests of the patient, even if this means overriding the views of relatives living in the same house with the patient. However, another frequently occurring community situation is when a relative is in danger of being exhausted by the demands of a caring task such as this case, again described by a district nurse:

'It's a situation where a daughter had very dutifully looked after both parents. The mother had Alzheimer's disease and in the last year father had developed cancer of the throat. She also had a daughter who at the age of 20 came off a motorbike and had a degree of paralysis of the lower pelvis. I literally walked in the door and she was tearing her hair out. Very tearful. Father was down the bottom of the garden, because he'd said some very unpleasant things: "Well you've got to move in here". I said, "I've got plenty of time because you're my last visit, and somehow I could sense when I came through the door that you really need to talk." I helped her to see the benefits of being able to go home at the end of the day. I asked her to consider whether or not she would feel more of a slave to her father. I didn't use those terms, but this is how I spoke. We talked about the value of having her own front door key. Did her father look upon her still as his little girl, or did he look upon her as a married woman with children? Had she asked her children how they felt about this? I did constantly sort of reassure her that throughout our conversation I was not going to judge her, whatever decision she made, "because I am a nurse and I have no right to encourage you or discourage you, that really is your decision".

She did say at the end of the day that there were a lot of things I was able to put before her that she hadn't even thought of because she had panicked. And after a few weeks she decided to stay independent, but accept more help. And she's never regretted it. In fact she's said on a number of occasions, "I don't know how to thank you for what you've done for me". And I said to her, "I've done nothing except all I did was to help you to see the whole problem, not just a section of it. You did it by yourself." She said, "Yes, but I couldn't have done it without you".'

So here the relative of the patient needed protecting from herself and from the demands of her father. Although the nurse formally remained neutral, it is clear that her intervention supported the carer's wish to continue living independently in her own home. It was a matter of helping the carer to preserve her own autonomy in the face of emotional blackmail from a member of her own family. In advocacy terms, the nurse empowered the daughter to make up her own mind and not to give way to the undue influence of her father. The nurse could defend her actions as being in the best interests not only of the daughter, but in the long term of the parents, since they helped to ensure the daughter did not exhaust herself both physically and emotionally.

Hospital care

Although advocacy with relatives in the community may seem complex, the power of patients and relatives living in their own homes appears to be a very important factor in determining outcomes. In contrast, situations involving relatives visiting patients in institutional settings change the balance of power drastically. This is shown most clearly in the case of hospitalised children. The legal position on consent to treatment broadly supports the right of parents of children under 16 years to give or withhold consent (Dimond 1993). However, this is not an absolute right. If the professionals believe that the parents' decision is against the best interests of the child, they may call upon the courts to intervene and determine the best course of action. In practice, however, many parents are left to feel that their ability to control even the everyday basics of what happens to their child is very limited once hospitalisation has occurred. The power of the professionals on their own territory is far-reaching. Because of this it is common for parents to see themselves as advocates for their child, supporting what they see as the best interests of the child, but leaving the ultimate decisions to the professionals.

Peter Callery (1995) conducted some research into parents' and nurses' participation in the care of hospitalised patients, with disturbing findings. He conducted conversational style interviews with parents of 24 children in their own homes during the weeks following discharge from a surgical ward of a children's hospital. In addition, there were approximately 125 hours of participant observation, principally of nursing handovers between shifts, plus interviews with 12 members of ward staff. Parents described being upset by involvement in some aspects of care, for example holding their child while a painful injection was given. One wonders whether parents felt guilty at exposing their child to pain or stress. Some of the parents identified themselves as in need of care during this difficult time, seeking support from within their own family but also from the nursing staff. The nurses agreed that they had some responsibilities towards the parents, particularly in teaching caring skills and offering health education, as well as counselling and general support. However the extent of this responsibility was not clear and led at least one nurse to talk about 'baby-sitting' the parents. Callery formed the view that care of parents was not usually planned on the basis of assessment of need, but it was left to individual nurses to respond to the immediate requirements of specific parents. The nurses felt that the demands of parents for time were unpredictable and presented them with problems in managing their work.

Callery (1995) found that judgements were made by the nurses about which parents were likely to present demands on their time, based on impressions and discussion about parents' rationality and intelligence. Nurses were particularly concerned about 'uptight' or 'anxious' parents. One nurse described the response of a mother to some technical equipment at the bedside:

'. . . it was unfortunate that she does have a phobia about the drips, machines, drains, and it was unfortunate that the once or twice when she did leave him something drastic happened while she was gone.'

Callery comments on the use of the term 'phobia', suggesting that the nurse thought there was something wrong with the mother, rather than a problem with the relationship between the nurses and the mother:

'Professionals are in a position to use diagnostic labels in a way that undermines the credibility of a mother and identifies her as the problem.' (Callery 1995)

The data from this ward suggest that the parents were expected to comply with the wishes of the professional staff. When parents questioned or refused to do what was required they were labelled as problems in themselves and in this way it became legitimate to treat them as not fully autonomous.

In a review of the literature on parental participation in care, Imelda Coyne (1995) cites numerous studies which broadly support Callery's conclusions and which emphasise parents' complaints that professional staff tend to provide too little information about a child's condition and treatment plan and about what is expected of the parents. Darbyshire (1992) studied the experiences of 30 parents who lived-in with their hospitalised child. They reported feeling uncertain about what was expected of them in relation to both their child's care and their personal behaviour. The parents felt under pressure to participate and establish themselves in the eyes of the professionals as 'good' parents, meaning cooperative, competent in basic child care and of good character. Brown & Ritchie (1990) concluded that nurses frequently lacked trust in parents and their ability to care for their children. They suggested that this lack of trust arose because the nurses felt threatened by increased parental participation in care.

Robinson (1972) found that parents became more assertive and less compliant the more experiences they had of being in hospital with their child or of dealing with the child's illness. The process appears very similar to the journey which Thorne & Robinson (1988) described for people with chronic illnesses, beginning with a naive faith in the professionals and all that they say or do, but ending either with distrust of all professionals or, more positively, a determination to work in partnership with selected professionals who showed respect for their autonomy. In Canada, Gibson (1995) studied mothers of children diagnosed as having chronic neurological problems. She found that the mothers experienced shock and disbelief when the diagnosis was first given, followed by delayed grief when the evidence of their own eyes showed them that their children were not developing at the same rate as others. The mothers then embarked on a quest for information in order to understand the situation. Initially they placed their trust in the professional staff who were providing advice and care and did not seek to influence or challenge treatment decisions. Because of their unfamiliarity with the situation, external sources of information were seen as authoritative. However, through caring for their child over a period of time, the mothers discovered the unique personal characteristics of the child and became experts on the child's responses through their constant monitoring of mood and behaviour. It was at this stage that they began to feel frustrated by the health care system which denied them information and by professionals who seemed to minimise their concerns and who failed to appreciate their growing expertise:

'Mothers described many kinds of irritations related to health care. Waiting was frustrating: waiting for the doctors or nurses to attend to the child – in the emergency department, in the hospital unit, or in the clinics; waiting for answers to questions; waiting for the child to heal or progress; or waiting for the child to have seizures when this was part of the diagnostic process. Travelling in and out of a large, congested city added to aggravations. Repeating the child's health history over and over as well as educating new residents was very irritating.' (Gibson 1995)

According to Gibson many mothers eventually came to realise that they knew their child better than anyone else and that they, rather than the professionals, were the experts on their own child's needs and responses. Once they were aware of this, they became confident in the role of advocate for the child, taking charge of the situation. They learned how to make the system work for them, for example by phoning specific members of the epilepsy team in advance of coming to the emergency department so that mother and child no longer had to wait and met professionals who were already familiar with the child. They also became much more persistent in the search for information, writing down their questions and requesting second opinions when dissatisfied. Some mothers enlisted the support of nurses as co-advocates because they believed that the doctors would more readily listen if the nurses were also putting forward their case. Gibson (1995) echoes Thorne & Robinson (1988) in saying that mothers wanted a partnership with the professionals, including respect for their knowledge of their children.

> 'All of the mothers reported that the hospital experience was very stressful. Mothers found it very difficult to have a sense of power in a setting where the practice model was hierarchical and medical needs were placed as primal. Yet the mothers, in their own way, initiated changes in their interactions with health care professionals and most became adept at making their voices heard. Clearly the mothers were the driving force for negotiations with health care professionals. Because they firmly believed that they knew their child best, they did not surrender their power passively to physicians or to anyone else.'
> (Gibson 1995)

Advocacy by relatives in a hospital situation usually takes the form of implied criticism of the care given by the professionals. The power struggle is not limited to one between parents of young children and the professionals. Relatives visiting a hospitalised adult are frequently the people who first complain about inadequacies of treatment or care on the patient's behalf. There is a sense in which it is safer for them to complain than for the patient to do so; the patient may fear victimisation or being labelled 'unpopular' (Stockwell 1984). However, just as in the home situation, relatives do not always act as altruistic advocates; they may have other motives, both conscious and unconscious.

A typical pressure situation is the case conference called when an elderly hospitalised patient is due to be discharged and the professionals are worried about the patient's ability to cope at home. The issue can turn into a power struggle where the patient wants either to return home or to live with relatives, while the family prefer nursing home care. Considerations of property ownership or nursing home fees may further undermine the credibility of family members as advocates for the needs of the patient.

Another point of tension concerns patients with terminal illnesses, where in the past medical staff have tended to use relatives as allies to support a policy of non-disclosure of a poor prognosis. Although the professionals appear to have become more committed to openness in recent years, some relatives advocate non-disclosure on the grounds that they know the patient intimately and believe that disclosure will lead to deep distress and depression. Sometimes this turns into a power struggle between doctors and nurses, with the medical staff typically favouring continued medical or surgical intervention and preservation of hope through limited disclosure and euphemism, while the nursing staff generally prefer openness and more palliative approaches to care. In this situation either group may seek to involve the relatives on their side to add weight to their views, as in the following account from an enrolled nurse:

'The patient was a very poorly man who vomited a large amount of blood and was referred to the surgical team by the medical team. He was seen by the surgical doctor on call and he decided he should take the patient to theatre. The patient had had a stroke recently and was dying slowly (he was unconscious at this stage). I discussed taking the patient to theatre with both teams. The medical team stated that once referred they really had to take the advice given. However, the patient's daughter had to sign the consent form. I telephoned her and informed her of the decisions made. She was horrified that her poorly father should be made to suffer further. I told her I agreed and advised her that she didn't have to sign the consent, the decision was hers. The daughter refused to sign the consent form, the patient didn't go to theatre and died comfortably a few days later.'

Taken as a whole the relationship between professionals and the relatives of patients is an uneasy one, frequently characterised by suspicion on both sides and leaving the sick person vulnerable to becoming a pawn in the midst of a power struggle. In recent years independent advocacy organisations have expanded their roles as objective advocates for patients, claiming to have no institutional or emotional axe to grind. The potential of these services is examined in the next chapter.

Summary of key points

- The place where a patient is living or being treated is usually the determining factor in the role of relatives in relation to advocacy
- If the family member is at home and being cared for by the relatives, their position power is fairly strong and the professionals may find

themselves cast in the weaker role of advocates trying to persuade the relatives of what is in the patient's best interests

- If the patient is in hospital or other institutional care, the roles are reversed; the relatives usually feel deprived of information and are not encouraged to participate in meaningful discussion of treatment or care
- It requires knowledge of the system and considerable determination for relatives to empower themselves; this can sometimes be achieved through advocacy alliances with members of staff, although relatives may also be enlisted by staff to support their own viewpoints
- When children suffer chronic health problems, the advocacy position of parents is strengthened over time by their in-depth knowledge of their own child and the gradual accumulation of information about the specific illness or disability
- Overall the literature suggests that the relationship between professionals and relatives is frequently one of rivalry in which both parties claim to be advocates as they struggle for control over the patient's care.

Chapter 11
Independent Advocacy

Some of the advocacy situations dealt with by health care professionals are essentially communication difficulties which can be speedily resolved once the client's wants are clearly understood by those in authority. However, more serious problems arise from issues of substance in which the client's wants are radically different from what the service providers regard as reasonable. Even with the best will in the world, confrontation is built into these situations and this is what makes it difficult for more junior professionals to speak up for their clients in the face of powerful opposition. This is where the availability of independent advocacy can help clients and shelter the professionals from risk by allowing them to make third party referrals.

In order to explore independent advocacy further, this chapter will examine in some detail the work of the only county-wide advocacy service in England – CALL or Citizen Advocacy Lincolnshire Link – drawing on information published by the organisation and the views of its manager, Muriel Ball. The need for an advocacy service in Lincolnshire was first identified by a group of parents of children with learning disabilities who wanted more independent support and forward planning than social services seemed able or willing to provide. A steering group was formed and advocacy partnerships established. CALL progressed to offer a generic service and charitable status was granted in 1989. Successful fund raising means that the organisation currently has five offices across the county. The development of the scheme has followed the sources of funding available, with special projects established to provide advocacy for the elderly in residential homes, for elderly people in rural communities, for young people between the ages of 18-25, and most recently for people with mental health problems.

CALL defines advocacy as verbal support or argument for a cause or policy. Thus an advocate is a person who supports or speaks in favour of a cause or another person. Independent or citizen advocacy is a one to one relationship between an unpaid advocate and a client or partner. The emphasis is on establishing a long-term relationship. Advocates help their partners by promoting their views and when appropriate speaking on their behalf to establish their rights. Advocates are people whose sole loyalty is to their partners, whose views and rights they commit to defend as vigorously as if they were their own. Because CALL advocates are ordinary people who voluntarily give their time, they can help to provide a link to community life for individuals who may have been excluded from some activities for many years. In addition to these long-term relationships, CALL volunteers also offer crisis advocacy for people who need the support of an independent advocate during a major change in their lives such as moving home or for a particular issue such as making a complaint. The ultimate goal is what CALL describes as exemplary advocacy, which is when the real needs of partners are met and they have the opportunity to lead enjoyable lives through effective and appropriate support. This can only be achieved if the partners remain in control of the advocacy they receive and wherever possible advocates work to promote self-advocacy. It also means giving partners access to whichever type of advocacy is needed at different times in their lives.

Partnerships

CALL is a generic advocacy service, but one which concentrates on helping people with disabilities whether arising from physical problems, learning difficulties, age or mental illness. These disabilities can easily lead to stigma and disadvantage with separation from friends and relatives and fewer choices or opportunities than are available to others. For example, an advocate was partnered with a young man who spent his days at a social education centre. The client was really interested in gardening and it was quite evident that this interest could not be fulfilled at the day centre, where the staff could not fully visualise his potential and in any case lacked the resources to support it. His advocate approached a local agricultural college and put forward a case for financial support for his partner. Eventually the young man was awarded a £3000 grant to support a course at the college. He successfully completed it and it proved a springboard to employment, independent living and later marriage.

Another example of successful advocacy concerned a young man of 19 who had been involved in an accident while out with friends. His injuries required only a short period of hospitalisation but had far-reaching effects, proving the last straw which threatened to overwhelm him. He had already spent most of his life in care, could hardly read or write and so was prone to misinterpreting situations or being misled by other people. After his accident he had given up his work training and was persuaded that because he was sick he did not have to sign on at the Job Centre and so received no income for several weeks. When he was referred to CALL he already owed several hundred pounds in rent, he had been relying on handouts for food and had been given one month to vacate his bedsit. His advocate helped him to present his case at the Job Centre and to get housing benefit, which allowed him to pay off his debts and avoid losing his home. The advocate also supported him in joining a basic education class, so improving his reading, writing and money management skills.

The nature of independent advocacy

These examples concentrate on the practical achievements of an independent advocacy service which has expertise in dealing with a wide range of external agencies. However, concentration on the more measurable outcomes obscures the gains which come from longer term relationships between volunteer advocates and their partners. As an experienced advocate, Muriel Ball, manager of CALL, argues that these relationships are different in quality from those that can be attained between professionals and patients. The difference arises from the greater independence of the advocate and the voluntary choice of both parties over the length and nature of the relationship. Muriel Ball was once a social worker and sums up her view of the advantages which independent advocacy offers:

> 'My feeling is that you cannot practise true advocacy when you have to work within an organisation that has policies. In the final analysis you are expected to follow the party line. As a social worker I had to adapt myself to my organisation or else get out, which is what I eventually chose to do. I think that professionals cannot do true advocacy and represent the individual in ways that make total change. The professionals have to leave on one side very great areas of conflict and are constantly at risk of being seen as no longer members of the team.'

This is not to say that CALL sees itself as anti-professional. The organisation seeks to work alongside the professionals and offer a service which adds benefit to what they provide. However, according to Muriel Ball it is hard to keep the professionals from becoming defensive:

> 'The problem for an advocacy scheme is to say we are not here to question your professionalism, but instead to speak on behalf of our partners and to put forward what they want. This means that we will

be seen at times to question the drugs, the placements, the benefits, the care plan and everything else. We can stand independently. This is why it is hard to sell independent advocacy to professionals. We try to work alongside the professionals, because there are some things we can do and some things they can do. We need them and they need us. For example we took up the case of a woman who for various reasons needed a shower fitted in her home and could not afford it herself. She was being pushed around from one part of social services to another and then on to the housing department, all with no effect. But with the help of her advocate she was able to make contact with four others who had similar problems. Then the advocate spoke on their behalf to all the local councillors and through this pressure they eventually succeeded in having showers put in. So you have to challenge the existing order sometimes. Certainly going round canvassing the local councillors is something the professionals cannot do if they hope to keep their jobs.'

CALL has also been involved where professional standards have slipped and where professionals have stood by while abuse has occurred. Muriel Ball was called in by social services when they realised that a woman going to a learning disabilities day centre regularly had unexplained bruises:

'They brought me in to act on behalf of the client independently. I discovered that she was the only one living in residential accommodation who was in a wheelchair and was being abused and hit by the residents because she was literally a sitting target for them to work out their own frustrations. The residential manager knew it was going on but took no action saying, "That's what it's like being here". I told the social worker my partner was to be moved and we went up one day, packed her things and moved her. It's made a huge difference to her. She can speak now, where she used to make animal noises. She has a much better quality of life.'

Referrals

Relatively few clients contact CALL on their own behalf. The reason is straightforward: the people who most need advocacy are the ones who are already disempowered and consequently have real difficulty in seeking it out for themselves. CALL therefore has specific written criteria for accepting referrals which include the following:

(1) The referral can either be a self referral or from a third party

(2)   We normally require there to be a 'presenting problem' or defined need; advocacy is not just a befriending service

(3)   The person referred generally must come within four main categories: learning difficulty, physical disability, mental illness or the elderly

(4)   The referral must be appropriate for advocacy. We are very willing to work jointly with other agencies, if this is deemed appropriate. CALL retains the right to refuse an inappropriate referral

(5)   The person referred must, as far as practicable, be aware of the reasons of the referral and the basic concept of advocacy

(6)   The person referred must be free to accept/refuse advocacy in general and the potential advocate for the partnership in particular, if they do not wish to have this facility

(7)   The prospective advocate is likewise free to refuse a potential partnership, if they personally do not feel it is appropriate or they consider that they would not have a comfortable relationship with the partner

(8)   Referrers must be aware that CALL will need to have specific information – which will be treated confidentially – regarding potential partners. This is particularly important if the lack of knowledge about a potential partner's physical or mental condition could put the advocate or the partner at risk during the normal course of the relationship

(9)   Referrers and potential partners should be aware that advocates are well briefed regarding matters of potential confidentiality

(10)   Confidences shared between partner and advocate during the course of the partnership must be respected.

The advocates

Anyone over the age of 18 is eligible to apply to become an advocate with CALL and currently the oldest is 77. They are very varied in life and work experience but are all required to supply two references, one professional and one personal. They may choose to work with a particular client group if they wish and the organisation currently has 70 advocates on its bank across the county. CALL volunteers must subscribe to seven principles of advocacy:

(1)   Act in the partner's best interest
(2)   Act in accordance with the partner's wishes
(3)   Keep the partner properly informed
(4)   Carry out instructions with diligence and competence

(5)   Act impartially and offer frank independent support
(6)   Advocates should maintain the rules of confidentiality
(7)   Act according to the guidelines of CALL.

Further guidance to prospective volunteers comes in the form of a definition which states that an advocate freely chooses to enter into a relationship with a person who is at risk of social exclusion, loss of rights and opportunities. Advocates find ways of understanding their partners' interests and represent them as if they were their own. Advocacy may involve helping to express an individual's concerns and aspirations, obtaining social, recreational, health and educational services and providing other practical and emotional support. Acceptance as an advocate depends on an initial interview with a coordinator, satisfactory references and successful completion of an induction programme, plus agreement to attend a 10-day initial training programme spread over approximately 12 months. Not all applicants are accepted.

Supervision

Advocates are accountable to named coordinators. These coordinators allocate partners as appropriate and provide regular one-to-one and group supervision. The coordinators themselves have regular monthly supervision at the centre. They are required to submit reports on activity and problems four days in advance of the meeting. In addition, regular top-up training and away days are organised each year. It is recognised that although technical knowledge of particular advocacy issues is not a requirement, there are advantages in having access to wide ranging areas of expertise. There is therefore a wider support network of expert advisers attached to CALL to help with the technicalities of problems involving mental health, learning disabilities and physical handicaps, plus support from a local group of solicitors for legal matters.

Independent advocacy in the health service

The tradition of independent advocacy is better established in areas concerned with social services than within the health service or independent health care sector. The professional, hierarchical structure of the NHS remains strong and this makes it difficult for external advocacy services to gain access. For CALL, a recent contact with a senior manager in a mental health trust has provided a starting point for a pilot advocacy service within a psychiatric in-patient unit. It is funded almost entirely within CALL's overall budget rather than through the health authority or the trust. It is too soon to evaluate the service.

Within primary care, GPs are independent contractors with no obligation to cooperate with independent advocates. In some cases the only option is to support the client in making a move to a more amenable GP practice.

Funding

The search for continuing funding is a constant problem for any advocacy service and CALL is no exception. It has no parent body with a central office that can take responsibility for raising money. Therefore some of CALL's local resources have to be spent on campaigning for financial support. Core funding is provided through an annual service agreement with the social services department, currently set at £55 000 per year but with no guarantee of continuity. Most additional funding comes from project monies rather than direct giving, since an advocacy service can hardly compete in the marketplace with other high profile charities. Like some other advocacy schemes, CALL was successful in a bid for Lottery monies for one of its projects. However, the funding on all Lottery projects is drip-fed, rather than given as a lump sum that would enable interest to be earned and genuine pump priming achieved. While this approach may safeguard the public purse, it also demands a vast amount of bureaucracy to compile the highly detailed and regular reports that the Lottery insists on to justify continuation of funding. In effect this means that a significant proportion of the Lottery funding has to be spent on additional administration to meet the funding criteria, rather than on the projects which money was originally intended to support!

For CALL some funding is agreed annually, other projects are funded for three years. This means that future planning is very difficult. With five offices across Lincolnshire CALL now employs 18 people, most of them part-time. Some are coordinators of the advocacy projects, paid at the rate each project allows. Others provide essential administrative support, generally at a minimal hourly rate. The volunteer advocates themselves are usually paid nothing and receive only limited expenses. For this advocacy service, as for most others, the price of independence is an uncertain financial future.

Conclusion

This chapter has highlighted the work of one independent advocacy service as an example of an organisation which is trying to provide a service that is complementary to the work of the professionals. The independence of the volunteers from the policies and employment rules which apply within health and social services means that they are not taking the same risks in speaking up for their clients which sympathetic professionals would be running. It means for example that they can challenge a psychiatrist's medication prescriptions on the basis that they are representing the wishes of their partner. In the same situation a nurse would run the risk of being seen as pursuing a personal agenda or as directly challenging the expert power of the psychiatrist. Similarly a volunteer advocate may safely appeal directly to members of a trust board or to local councillors, where a professional employee would be open to criticism for trying to bypass the organisation's chain of authority.

Balancing these advantages are the problems of limited funding and denial of access to the places where potential clients are located. A reliance on project monies means that independent advocacy services have to concentrate their efforts on specific groups of people, defined as being in need by the agencies which are funding the projects. With social workers now offering more of a brokerage service than the direct support and care which they used to give, the advocacy needs of people living in the community appear to have become greater in recent years. However, independent advocacy has been shown to work very effectively alongside advocacy by professionals, setting the same high standards for the quality of its services and making the same use of sound and regular supervision.

Summary of key points

- Independent advocacy schemes are expanding their role and are no longer restricted to working with people with learning disabilities
- They tend to define advocacy as a long-term relationship with a partner, with self-advocacy as their ideal aim
- They can challenge authority more vigorously and in a more political way than most professionals
- The price of their independence is a constant struggle to maintain adequate funding.

Chapter 12
Supervision

The words and actions of advocates affect the lives of others, both clients and colleagues. Some form of supervision of how they work is essential so that clients have an assurance of safe practice. It also provides a vital support for the advocates themselves, since advocacy can be work that is both stressful and lonely. In the words of John Southgate, 'An advocate needs an advocate' (Teasdale 1991). This in fact is just another way of describing supervision, a notion which began in psychotherapy as a way of helping and supporting new therapists. Because of the intensely personal nature of psychotherapy, therapists usually worked alone with their clients. Therefore they began taking time outside their casework to describe and reflect on their work in the presence of a more experienced therapist or supervisor. On some occasions supervisors would advise therapists about what they should or should not do with their clients. At other times, they would draw on their own experience to teach the therapists new techniques. However, most of the time would be spent listening and giving support to the therapists in their emotionally demanding work. It is easy to see how advocates can benefit from similar support by establishing formal supervision arrangements.

Different options in supervision

The most frequently used form of supervision is the one-to-one session away from patients or clients. Typically it lasts for about one hour and centres on discussion of the detail of patient or client advocacy. In some cases, the supervisor is a more experienced advocate who is entirely concerned with supporting and helping a less experienced colleague. Alternatively, it may be a meeting between two colleagues who take it in turns to describe key issues and who supervise each other. This approach is often called 'peer' supervision.

Group supervision is also popular, particularly within teams working with similar types of patients or clients. Group sessions tend to

113

require more time than one-to-one because of the number of people contributing. Some groups have an outside expert to lead them. This person may be a technical expert in the topic being discussed but more usually is an expert in running therapeutic groups. Here the supervisor sets the agenda for the meeting in discussion with the group, organises the time for as many people to contribute as possible, enforces ground rules to promote good listening and constructive commentating, and then summarises key learning points at the end. An alternative is a peer group, where there is no formal leader or where leadership alternates from meeting to meeting. The value of group supervision is that it allows individuals to sound-out a group of colleagues on their clinical issues, providing powerful criticism or strong support for different courses of action. The drawbacks are the limited amount of time for each individual and the risk that criticism may move from constructive to destructive.

Some supervision arrangements use diary records produced by supervisees (Love 1996a). The aim is to capture day-to-day events while their impact is still fresh, then to reflect on them at leisure in the presence of a supervisor. This form of supervision requires a great deal of discipline from the supervisee, but can be particularly valuable in revealing repeated patterns of behaviour among apparently diverse advocacy situations. Tape or video recordings can also be used and they are particularly valuable for focusing on interpersonal skills. They can only be made with the permission of clients and many advocates are reluctant to ask because they imagine the recording apparatus will be off-putting. However, video cameras have reduced in size and small tape recorders are unobtrusive. It is amazing how much can be learned from recordings and they are a great help to supervisors in bringing to life the reality of everyday advocacy. The following tape recorded dialogue illustrates one-to-one supervision in advocacy involving a nurse who has regular clinical supervision with a more experienced colleague:

SUPERVISOR: 'Tell me about the advocacy incident you mentioned earlier.'

ADVOCATE: 'Well I don't know if I'd really call it advocacy – failed advocacy maybe. You see this young girl was attending the clinic and she didn't want to be seen by a particular doctor that she'd met before and who she felt wasn't sympathetic to her. But the duty doctor insisted on calling in this particular colleague who shouted at the patient and reduced her to tears about her request. I was totally shocked at what happened and unfortunately I did nothing during the incident, though I think now that I should have done. Instead I offered support to the patient afterwards, apologised for how the situation had been handled and gave her time in private to compose herself. But I felt afterwards I'd let her down.'

SUPERVISOR: 'Can you say what you felt you should have done?'

ADVOCATE: 'Well, I think I should have spoken to the doctor there and then. In fact I chose not to confront this doctor because she is well known for shouting when challenged and this wouldn't have enhanced the situation, even though that's what I felt like doing at an emotional level. Instead I decided that the patient's best interests would be served by talking to my manager who I knew would be supportive to the patient and who I hoped would discuss the situation with the medical staff.'

SUPERVISOR: 'So it sounds as though you very quickly thought about the risks of speaking up directly on behalf of the patient but judged that this would only make the situation worse – is that right?'

ADVOCATE: 'Yes, I suppose I did think it out, or maybe I just acted that way instinctively. It all happened very quickly.'

SUPERVISOR: 'So did you speak to your manager about the doctor shouting at the patient?'

ADVOCATE: 'Yes I did, but my manager wasn't willing to do anything about it and would not support me in directly questioning the medical staff about it. I felt let down because they were left unchallenged about their behaviour.'

SUPERVISOR: 'I can understand you feeling let down. It's a real problem for an advocate when more senior people in the organisation won't support them. I often think in this situation you have to come back to your client and see whether they're willing to speak up for themselves.'

ADVOCATE: 'In fact that's what I did. I explained to her the choices she had about future attendances at the clinic, or going to another clinic, or having a word with her GP. I also told her that she had a right to complain if she wanted and explained the complaints procedure. She thought about it but in the end decided she didn't want to do anything, although she didn't have a good word to say about any of the medical staff. I was pleased that she did return as planned next time and completed the tests as prescribed. I think at least she felt that I supported her.'

SUPERVISOR: 'Which I also think you did. You helped her to understand her rights. And in the end it's down to the clients to choose for themselves. Without their backing you can't do any more. Would you agree with that?'

ADVOCATE: 'Yes, I think I feel a bit more at ease with myself after talking it out like this. I suppose I took that particular incident as far as I could, but I can see myself having to confront that doctor in the future if something similar happens.'

SUPERVISOR: 'I wonder, is that something you can take up now with your manager. I don't mean ask his advice, but explain what you did for this client as you've just explained it to me and then tell him that in a similar situation in the future you would want to intervene earlier and more directly with the doctor.'

ADVOCATE: 'I suppose that's not a bad idea. At least I could sound my manager out to see if I could count on his support.'

SUPERVISOR: 'Yes, and it would also mean that if the doctor put in a counter-claim in the future you could say that there was a history of problems with this particular doctor and your manager would have to admit that you had already brought an incident to his attention.'

ADVOCATE: 'It sounds a bit devious, but I can see the sense in it.'

Supervision like this can have three main functions, described by Proctor (1991) as 'normative, formative and restorative' (Fig. 12.1). Normative supervision is best understood as a supervisor giving advice or making suggestions with an emphasis on improving the quality of an advocate's work. The final suggestion by the supervisor in the example above about going back to the manager could be regarded as a tentatively normative intervention. In contrast, formative supervision means learning about advocacy either from direct teaching by

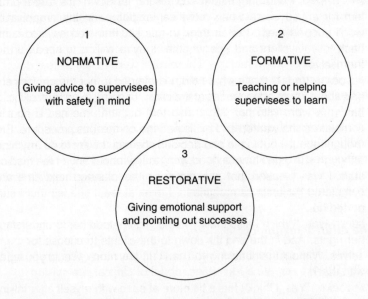

Fig. 12.1   The three functions of supervision (from Proctor 1991).

the supervisor or through a more facilitative approach involving suggestions about suitable study materials, or challenging questions that promote self awareness and reflection. It is helpful in formative supervision if the supervisor has greater knowledge or experience of some aspects of the work than the supervisee. The supervisor in the example asked the supervisee what more she thought she could have done in the situation. This was essentially formative, challenging her to examine her own practice and to learn from it for the future. Finally, restorative supervision means sharing some of the stresses and strains of advocacy with a knowledgeable and empathic listener, within an agreed contract of confidentiality. The example above contains many restorative elements, with the supervisor essentially helping the advocate to notice the things she did well and not to punish herself unreasonably over the outcome.

Models of supervision

A question often asked by supervisees is how they can judge for themselves the quality of the supervision they are receiving. One answer is that the best forms of supervision promote reflection, encouraging supervisees to stop and think about things for themselves. The most influential writer on this topic has been Donald Schon (1983). He studied the ways professionals take decisions and found similarities between people working in fields as different as medicine, architecture and the law. In these complex activities, practitioners did not apply rules directly from the text books. Instead they linked knowledge from reading with practical understanding from past experience and worked out their own rules for decision-making. These rules were rarely written down or made conscious, they simply developed over time as part and parcel of becoming an experienced professional. Schon also noticed that experienced professionals experimented in their practice. They tried out new ways of doing things, took note of the outcomes and then modified their practice as a result. Schon coined the name of 'reflective practice' for this process of developing rules for decision-making from both academic knowledge and experience, then testing them out further through informal experimentation.

The adult learning cycle

Schon's ideas can be linked with the adult learning cycle proposed by Kolb (1984) to create a four-stage model of clinical supervision:

(1) Adults accumulate practical experience at work, some of which

worries or puzzles them and provides a starting point for new learning

(2) They reflect on these events afterwards, thinking them over or talking about them to others; they may go to written sources of information at this stage to help them to increase their understanding of what has happened

(3) Then they try to encapsulate their learning into resolutions for the future

(4) Finally they attempt to put their resolutions into practice as events permit and so the learning cycle returns to stage one.

Using the adult learning cycle as a supervisee, one begins with advocacy experience, captured through reflection in action as events occur during a busy working day. Then within the supervision session itself, selected events are recalled and described to the supervisor or supervision group. Discussion follows in which the supervisee reflects on what happened, listens to suggestions and comments and then draws new meaning from the clinical events. This new meaning should lead to action. It may be a change in advocacy practice, a decision to test out new ways of working, or a confirmation of good practice and a renewed determination to continue as before. It is by completing the cycle, bringing it back to renewed practical work, that the supervisee becomes a better advocate.

The learning cycle also guides the supervisor. The supervision session actually begins at stage two and the model reminds the supervisor to encourage the practitioner to describe events selected from advocacy experience (stage one) in as much detail as will make them understandable. Listening with attention is required to help the supervisee feel safe in recalling events in the presence of the supervisor or supervision group. At stage three, careful questioning may help the advocate to reflect on the meaning of events. For example, questions such as, 'How did you feel about that at the time? Do you still feel the same, or have things changed now?' Here the supervisor is trying to encourage the advocate to reflect on the emotional content of a particular event, using a comparison between now and the past to stimulate new learning. The techniques are the same as those used in many forms of counselling when the counsellor is trying to encourage the client to achieve a deeper level of understanding of what has happened. Finally, in stage four the supervisor may summarise what has been said and then ask the supervisee to state a plan of action for the future, for example, 'Having thought about it, is there anything you will do differently in the future?' or 'You've said you need to learn more about this, so what will be your first step?'

Preparing to be supervised

To get the most out of supervision it is essential to prepare beforehand. The ideal situation is to work in an organisation which promotes a variety of approaches to supervision, so that supervisees have real choice. However, even if options are severely restricted, supervisees should at least give some thought to what is available and whether or not it will meet their needs. One consideration is whether it is better to go for individual or group supervision. Individual supervision makes it easier to talk about difficult or emotionally charged issues, provided that a trusting relationship can be built up with the supervisor. It usually gives supervisees more time to present issues than can be found within group supervision. On the other hand, group supervision may offer the opportunity to hear a wide variety of feedback and can be very valuable in promoting good teamwork.

Both forms of supervision may use expert supervisors or may be established with peers or colleagues. With individual supervision, advocates may wish to seek supervision from a more experienced member of staff in their own work area, or they may choose to go to an expert who works in a different location in search of greater objectivity and perhaps confidentiality. On the other hand, some advocates may prefer to choose a peer, sharing supervision with someone they know and trust as an equal, again either involving someone from their own team or from outside. In group supervision, the usual choice is between having an expert to lead the sessions or keeping them entirely in-house and organising them as a group of colleagues. Many organisations now regard clinical supervision as essential for professional staff and see it as an integral part of their contract, supporting supervision within work time provided the parties involved consult over timing and frequency. Part of these sessions may be used for discussion of advocacy work and part for other clinical issues of importance. However, some professionals may prefer to arrange supervision in their own time as a way of ensuring their professional autonomy and confidentiality.

Negotiating the contract

At the start of supervision it is important to negotiate a contract, and this applies to both individual and group supervision. Negotiations are two-way and most supervisors will have views on what should be included, but it is important for supervisees to get their own position clear before starting to negotiate. One element of a contract will be the function of supervision, such as whether the emphasis is on the normative, formative or restorative functions. For example, a newly qualified professional or a newly recruited independent advocate may seek a certain degree of normative supervision. This would mean the supervisor pointing out mistakes or advising in a fairly directive way how to handle particular advocacy issues. Supervision for new advocates must also contain strong formative elements, with the supervisor at times teaching directly and at other times suggesting reading material or other ways of learning. In this situation the relationship is not equal in terms of knowledge and skills, although it should be equal in terms of mutual respect.

The advocate will be looking for a supervisor who has greater knowledge and experience and yet who is able to impart these without being overpowering or authoritarian. This issue of the balance of power within a supervisory relationship is an important consideration. Thus a more experienced advocate may not want any strong normative or formative elements. Instead the emphasis may be on the restorative function – looking for someone to share the stresses and strains of everyday advocacy. In this case a peer may be more appropriate than an expert supervisor, since an equal relationship in terms of knowledge and skills is required. A group can also be very supportive provided the group dynamics are competently handled. However, pressure of work means it can prove hard to maintain attendances over more than a limited number of sessions.

Content

The content or model of supervision should also be agreed explicitly at the start. In group supervision the content or model must be agreed by everyone. Groups frequently restrict the subject matter more than in individual supervision and concentrate on a limited range of clinical issues which affect all members. Another matter worth being particularly clear about is the boundary between clinical supervision and personal counselling. Many advocacy situations will arouse strong emotions and it is perfectly legitimate to bring these into supervision. However, sometimes the emotions attached to advocacy work are symptoms of a deeper level of distress in the advocate's personal life and relationships. A different contract is required for counselling in these situations, and the person chosen as an advocacy supervisor may not be the best choice for more personal counselling; indeed the supervisor may be unable to give the time and emotional commitment required in counselling. Therefore it is useful if the supervisor is given permission to point out when this boundary is in danger of being crossed, without this destroying the supervisory relationship.

Figure 12.2 shows an overview of supervision.

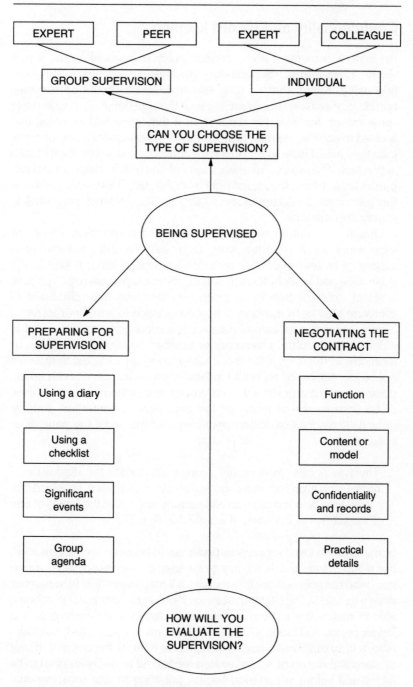

Fig. 12.2 Overview of supervision.

Confidentiality and record keeping

An explicit agreement about confidentiality is essential in any supervisory relationship. Supervisees generally want complete confidentiality, asking that nothing said in sessions should be repeated outside. Supervisors usually seek to limit the confidentiality guarantee to some extent, for example stating that if they were told anything that seemed to contravene their professional or organisational code of ethics then they would have to act on it if the supervisee were unwilling to take action first. The essence of any agreement on confidentiality is that both parties know where they stand right from the start. This makes it safe for the supervisee to accept responsibility for the material presented in supervision sessions.

Options for written records are many and varied. Supervisees or supervisors (or both) may write their own records. Sometimes a supervisor writes a brief open record in a notebook which is kept by the supervisee and brought to each session. Some supervision groups have a set of notes written by a group secretary and then circulated to everyone after each meeting. It is good practice to agree *not* to name clients, colleagues or clinical areas during supervision sessions, and in written records to use nicknames or numbers to identify individuals or locations. In this way, if the records happened to be mislaid they would not be identifiable by an outsider. Nevertheless, if supervision is taking place in work time or using work premises, any written records are likely to be seen as the property of the employing organisation and are potentially disclosable documents in legal actions involving patients or colleagues:

> 'The courts can, in personal injury cases, order the disclosure of information even before a court action has been started, provided that it is likely to be relevant to an issue arising and it is in the hands of one of the parties to the case.' (Dimond 1993, p.38)

Some advocates and supervisors prefer not to keep written records at all. For a supervisee who is receiving one-to-one supervision and a supervisor who has only one or two supervisees it may be possible to remember what was said in the previous session. However, there is value in being able to review the pattern of supervision topics and decisions over a longer period and this is where written records are particularly valuable. Also, a busy supervisor may be quite unable to recall the content of past sessions without some sort of written record. All these issues need to be negotiated before supervision begins, adhering to any organisational policies on supervision and record keeping.

Practical details

Where will supervision take place? It needs to be somewhere private and if group supervision is taking place the room must be large enough to hold the group comfortably. When will it take place, how long will it last and how frequently will sessions be held? There are no rules about frequency. Some groups meet weekly, some individual sessions take place at two-monthly intervals – it all depends on the needs of the advocate and the time that the supervisor is willing to make available. Another question is when will supervision cease? If neglected, this can lead to embarrassment later on. It is perfectly possible to have a one-off supervision session to deal with a particular problem and no more. If ongoing supervision is sought, it is a good idea to agree a limited number of sessions and then renegotiate if required. Supervision continuing without end can become a burden on all parties. For groups, agreement on a fixed number of sessions may help to keep up attendance. If participants know there are just six sessions at monthly intervals and then the group will stop, they are more likely to attend frequently and purposefully than if they believe they can pick up the group at any time in the future.

Preparing for sessions

Given the time and money which supervision costs, it is important to make the best use of each session. Once the contract has been agreed, the main work in preparation is to decide on the issues to be discussed. Essentially this is the prerogative of the supervisee, in the same way that in counselling it is the client who decides what to talk about. The model of supervision will determine the main topics, but usually most of the time is spent talking about casework, either focusing on particular clients or groups of clients, or raising related issues concerning colleagues or other professionals. The aim for the supervisee is to recall and prepare to describe important situations so that deeper level reflection and a move towards action can take place during the session itself.

A more detailed model of supervision which brings out additional aspects of the process has been developed by Dexter and Russell (1995). This model places the patient or client at the centre of supervision and divides the content of supervision sessions into five key issues:

(1) Mutual contracting
(2) Casework discussion
(3) Goal setting

(4)   Resources and planning
(5)   Training and information giving.

Mutual contracting means formalising supervision by agreeing in advance the nature of the relationship, the limits of confidentiality and the practicalities of how sessions will run. Casework discussion follows the same process as in the adult learning cycle, but Dexter and Russell also emphasise that it is legitimate to discuss the strengths and talents of supervisees as well as any personal or interpersonal issues which affect the advocacy or the supervision process. For example, personal issues may be stirred up as a result of advocates identifying closely with particular clients. Also, it is not unusual for supervision sessions to have to deal in great depth with interpersonal issues concerning colleagues, or general issues concerning the inadequacies of the organisations within which the advocates work. Goal setting as used by Dexter and Russell means discussing the types of goal which it is appropriate to agree with particular clients, to emphasise the importance of commitment from clients to the advocacy process. It can also be used as a reminder from time to time to review the advocate's own personal and professional goals. Discussion of resources and planning involves general caseload management, time management, budgetary constraints, etc. – the whole range of managerial issues which ultimately affect advocates' availability to clients. Finally, training and information-giving are concerned with the individual development of the advocate and may be linked with personal goals.

This model explicitly acknowledges that supervision may be individual or group and may include involvement of peers as opposed to expert supervisors. It also mentions self as a reminder of the importance of going over events in one's own mind rather than talking about them to someone else. Finally, the model suggests that many of the preconditions for a supervisory relationship are the same as those within counselling, requiring the creation of an atmosphere of trust which promotes good listening, empathy, mutual respect and honesty. Whichever model is chosen, the use of supervision needs to be taught and emphasised from the very start of an advocate's work, being built into an advocacy training curriculum.

Summary of key points

- Supervision is essential to safeguard clients and support advocates
- It may be normative, formative or restorative
- The adult learning cycle provides a straightforward model

- Advocates and supervisors need to negotiate a contract which includes the content of sessions, confidentiality and record keeping, and practical issues
- An advocate needs an advocate.

Chapter 13
An Advocacy Curriculum

Advocacy can be a risky business for all concerned and is certainly not something to be undertaken lightly. However, all health care professionals will at times act as advocates for patients and clients. Meanwhile, independent advocacy organisations are recruiting volunteers to work with wider groups of clients than ever before. If all these people are to be safe and effective advocates, they need education and training to help them meet the demands of the role. This chapter presents some ideas for inclusion in an advocacy curriculum, which could be used by teachers in the design of their programmes or by individual advocates in order to evaluate their current level of competence. It is not intended to be prescriptive but aims to cut out some of the basic work in curriculum design and allow users to concentrate on refining programmes to meet the needs of the target group.

Some initial work on competence in advocacy has already been undertaken by the National Council for Vocational Qualifications, using the dictionary definition of 'speaking on behalf of another, one who pleads the cause of another, an intercessor or defender'. The Council has drawn up advocacy standards for support workers who are completing a National Vocational Qualification (NVQ). Unit Z2 specifies criteria for a support worker to help a health care professional and contribute to advocacy for a patient or client. The unit recognises that advocacy may be long-term or short-term and that clients may vary widely in their ability to make decisions about what they want from advocacy. It divides advocacy into four elements:

Z2a Enable clients to establish their need for advocacy
Z2b Enable the client to obtain an advocate
Z2c Act as an advocate on a client's behalf
Z2d Enable the client to assess the effects of advocacy.

Element Z2a emphasises promoting choice and participation by the client through active listening, clear explaining and being prepared to seek advice or help from others. The section on underpinning knowledge brings out the limits of the support worker's role, the advantages and disadvantages of advocacy for clients, confidentiality and other legal issues, and methods of empowering clients in decision-making.

Element Z2b is concerned with helping clients to think through what they want and do not want from advocacy. It deals with making an initial contact with an advocate; with briefing an advocate on the client's rights and responsibilities and the advocate's role in supporting these; with introducing advocate and client; and with recording information relating to the advocacy. The knowledge base includes a value judgement about the advantages of the client choosing an independent advocate rather than a relative or friend, plus methods of referral.

Element Z2c deals with situations where support workers act as advocates on behalf of clients. The performance criteria build in safeguards for clients based on clear identification of what clients want, anticipation of any potential conflicts of interest, decision-making which is consistent with clients' values and needs, and a readiness to seek advice and offer other forms of advocacy if necessary. The knowledge base is similar to that for Element Z2b.

Element Z2d concentrates on monitoring and evaluating advocacy, particularly from the client's point of view. It recognises the support worker's role in raising any concerns about the effectiveness of advocacy with the client and seeking additional advice if required. The outcomes to be monitored are listed as representation of clients' values, needs, preferences, interests and rights, together with effectiveness, efficiency and clients' feelings about the process overall. The underpinning knowledge emphasises that outcomes should be assessed against the goals agreed at the start of advocacy.

It would be possible to extend this NVQ approach for support workers to specify higher level competences for health care professionals or for independent advocates who were to be involved in longer term working with clients. The advocacy flowchart in Fig. 4.1 could form the basis for these extended units and elements of competence. However, the NVQ approach functions more as an assessment tool than as a teaching or learning aid. It has also been found to need improvement because in the past it has placed too little emphasis on the knowledge base required to perform complex activities (NCVQ 1997). Indeed, by reducing activities into the minute detail of their component parts, an NVQ approach may appear rather mechanistic and unrelated to the complex and swiftly changing realities of everyday advocacy. Also, an emphasis on assessment of competence can promote defensive practices in which trainee advocates concentrate on finding evidence for what they believe they are already doing well, rather than seeking out new knowledge or skills.

On the positive side, the emphasis in NVQs on providing practical evidence of competence (rather than theoretical discussion) is one which can be transferred into a more traditional curriculum by specifying behavioural objectives at the start of the design process and then by seriously attempting to assess performance evidence as well as knowledge.

In higher education, the more familiar approach to curriculum development is to specify behavioural objectives (frequently called outcomes) rather than to go into the level of detail required by NVQ-style written competence statements. Behavioural objectives specify what a trainee advocate should be able say or do at the end of a period of learning and they are therefore particularly helpful for tutors who are designing classroom programmes. For example, a general purpose set of objectives might be developed out of the advocacy flowchart, as shown in Table 13.1. Another advantage of behavioural objectives over competences is that they are shorter and easier to understand. This does mean that they lack detail, but any single objective can be expanded as required. Thus, objectives seven and eight in Table 13.1 describe complex activities which might usefully be dealt with in greater depth. Examples of these expanded objectives are shown in Table 13.2.

Teaching plans

A teaching plan for trainee advocates will depend very much on the previous experience of the learners and on the amount of time which can reasonably be given to such a programme. Some examples will be

Table 13.1 General advocacy objectives.

---

(1) Describe the difference between 'needs' and 'wants' in advocacy.
(2) Assess whether or not different clients can identify their own wants.
(3) Contribute to a discussion of when one can reasonably assume clients' wants.
(4) Contribute to a debate about moral justifications for refusing to undertake advocacy.
(5) Identify the main risks arising from different forms of advocacy and how they can be eliminated or minimised.
(6) Assess whether or not different clients can self-advocate with help.
(7) Demonstrate skills in empowering clients to self-advocate.
(8) Demonstrate skills in undertaking advocacy on behalf of clients.
(9) Identify independent sources of advocacy and describe when and how to refer clients.
(10) Accept and use supervision to develop as an advocate.

Table 13.2 Expanded objectives.

Empowerment for self-advocacy
(1) Identify the types of knowledge clients will require in order to self-advocate.
(2) Supply information to clients in ways they understand.
(3) Help clients to find out additional information for themselves.
(4) Use counselling skills to support clients in making informed choices.
(5) Assist clients in rehearsing questions and statements to prepare to self-advocate.
(6) Identify ways of preparing the ground for self-advocacy.
(7) Demonstrate skills in supporting clients engaged in self-advocacy.

External advocacy
(1) Justify the choice of advocacy over empowerment for specific clients.
(2) Identify the information required to speak out as an advocate for specific clients.
(3) Agree a formal or informal advocacy contract with clients.
(4) Identify potential risks in advocacy for specific clients and specify how these risks can be eliminated or minimised.
(5) Analyse the balance of power in specific advocacy situations and use this to plan advocacy.
(6) Demonstrate assertive skills in undertaking advocacy on behalf of clients.

given here, based on a university-style 100-hour module comprising four days (24 hours) classroom teaching, an equivalent amount of time for guided study based mainly around directed reading and assuming about eight days (52 hours approximately) in collecting and recording practical experience. This module could be expanded or reduced, depending on the constraints affecting particular programmes. Programmes could also be run using full-day sessions as shown here, or split into smaller units, although with practical skills such as those involved in advocacy it is important to intersperse classroom work with practical experience. Therefore it would probably be less effective to run the module as a straight four-day block than as a series of study sessions. The only exception might be when dealing with carefully-prepared advocates who already have considerable knowledge and experience to draw on.

It is good practice in an advocacy course to make use of some external speakers whose points of view about advocacy may differ from those of the resident tutor. If the course is being run for health care professionals, ideal choices would include independent advocates, and speakers from social services and organisations such as the Citizens Advice Bureau. On a course for independent advocates, it would be valuable to invite relevant health care professionals to speak. In addition, a complaints officer from a hospital or a member of the community health council could contribute a different viewpoint. The remainder of this chapter shows sample teaching plans for each of the four days of a course. Different programme organisers will expand or reduce particular sections of the course, but the aim is to provide an introduction for new advocates which can be followed up in continuing education. The teaching plans are shown without detailed timings and breaks, since these will depend on the size of the group and facilities available.

Day 1

Aims

To provide a general introduction to advocacy in health care.

Objectives

At the end of the day, each participant will be able to do the following:

(1) Explain the advocacy flowchart (Fig. 4.1)
(2) Analyse a case study example using the flowchart
(3) Identify personal learning needs in advocacy.

Teaching plan

Morning

- Introductions and explanation of the design of the programme as a whole. Participants to explain their motivation in studying advocacy.
- Tutor to give examples of advocacy from personal experience in order to illustrate the nature of advocacy in health care.
- Tutor to offer a definition of advocacy and brief explanation of it, without at this stage going into the detail of the advocacy flowchart.
- Participants to contribute to a discussion of the extent to which their understanding and experience of advocacy matches the examples given by the tutor. The discussion may usefully be broadened to take in the issue of why patients in a caring health care system should need advocacy at all.
- Participants to recall and write down personal examples of advocacy from any context, whether as advocates or clients, and whether health care or not.

- Divide into groups of 4–6 people and ask participants to share their examples with group members. When all examples have been explained and discussed, group members to list what they have learned about advocacy from the discussion, plus any questions for the tutor. Also ask group members to select one example which is particularly clearcut to be repeated to the larger group.
- Everyone to return to large group, take the example from each small group in turn and deal with each group's summary of what they have learned and any questions. Use this exercise to evaluate the general level of understanding of advocacy within the group and to establish any aspects which will need particular attention during the rest of the programme.

Afternoon

- Give each participant a copy of the advocacy flowchart and explain it in detail. If possible, refer to the examples from group members to illustrate key points. Allow for debate about the flowchart, presenting it as a tool for learning rather than the one correct prescription for advocacy.
- Prepare in advance some examples of advocacy (or use examples from the next chapter) which will illustrate the main points of the flowchart. Divide back into small groups of 4–6 people and ask groups to analyse one different example each, following the flowchart. One group member should summarise the discussion, perhaps producing a flipchart sheet which shows the nature of the analysis. Return to one large group and examine each flipchart in turn. Allow members of other groups to comment and criticise, with the aim of reinforcing understanding of the flowchart and correcting any misunderstandings.
- Prepare in advance a display of patient information leaflets relevant to the types of advocacy which group members will be undertaking. Allow group members to browse through the leaflets, asking them to view them from the perspective of the patient groups at which they are aimed. Ask group members to comment on the extent to which the leaflets might meet their information and empowerment needs and to suggest improvements where possible.
- Ask participants to come to the next session prepared to report on how they have worked with at least two patients/clients in order to identify their *wants* as opposed to *needs* from the health and social care system. Also suggest relevant reading on ethical issues concerned with autonomy and beneficence in health care.

Day 2

Aims

To explore ethics, skills and risks related to advocacy, particularly in empowerment.

Objectives

At the end of the day each participant will be able to do the following:

(1) Identify the ethical issues which may arise in advocacy
(2) Explain the importance of identifying wants rather than ascribing needs in advocacy
(3) Identify some of the most common risks in advocacy
(4) Practise skills in empowering patients.

Teaching plan

Morning

- Tutor to give an initial lecture on ethical issues in advocacy, explaining key principles such as autonomy, beneficence, non-maleficence and justice (see Beauchamp & Childress 1979 for a detailed discussion). Use discussion to help individuals work out their initial position on issues such as: when one person's autonomy restricts the freedoms of another; when a patient seeks advocacy in a cause which the potential advocate does not support; when a powerful clinician claims that beneficence or non-maleficence should take priority over respect for autonomy etc.
- Either in small groups or in one large group, ask participants to describe their practical examples of working with patients/clients to identify their wants. Encourage group members to identify good techniques or skills employed. Use the examples to reinforce the distinction between needs and wants and to emphasise the importance of the latter. If appropriate, link examples with the preceding discussion on ethics.
- Use brainstorming either in small groups or in one large group to identify the main risks associated with advocacy. It may be useful to get groups to identify three categories of risk: to the patient; to the advocate; to colleagues and people in power.

Afternoon

- Tutor to introduce the theme of empowerment or self-advocacy. It may be useful to divide it into two elements:

  (1) Helping patients to acquire information and make decisions
  (2) Supporting and preparing the ground for them to speak up for themselves.

- Tutor to demonstrate information-giving and counselling skills in a role play. Seek feedback identifying the skills and techniques used and commenting on anything the advocate could have done better. Then divide group members into threesomes and ask them to role play similar situations with one observer to comment on the performance of the advocate. It may be best to let the advocates take the situation as they find it, but to give each patient a briefing on a card of the key points of concern.
- If possible use an external speaker to give a short session on the types of information about health-related issues which advocates may need to seek out.
- Tutor to use case studies to illustrate the ways advocates can support or prepare the ground to help patients speak out for themselves.
- Ask group members to come to the next session prepared to present a case study account of occasions when they have tried to empower patients, either successfully or unsuccessfully. Suggest background reading on the risks of advocacy.

Day 3

Aims

To introduce supervision and review skills and risks related to speaking out on behalf of patients.

Objectives

At the end of the day, each participant will be able to do the following:

(1) Discuss empowerment and its limits
(2) Accept supervision and learn from it
(3) Identify the skills used in advocacy when this means speaking out on behalf of patients
(4) Identify ways of eliminating or minimising risks arising from advocacy.

Morning

- Tutor to explain the value of supervision in advocacy. Explain a simple model of supervision and then invite group members to volunteer to present their homework examples of empowerment in a supervision session with the tutor as supervisor. After one or two sessions with discussion, divide into pairs and run a peer-supervision session. Tutor and volunteer group members may move between pairs, commenting on their observations.
- Tutor to remind group members of the essentials of advocacy, using the word in its narrow sense to mean speaking out on behalf of patients. Identify the situations in which it is appropriate to use advocacy. Allow group members to list some of the risks associated with it. Briefly explain the different types of power and how they may affect advocacy situations.
- Invite an external speaker with experience in advocacy to give some examples and promote discussion.

Afternoon

- Tutor to set up a case conference or similar role play involving advocacy. Invite one participant to be the advocate for a patient who is not present and others to play appropriate parts. This role play needs more detailed briefing than the others, but appropriate case study material can be found in Chapter 14 of this book. Tutor and remaining group members to observe. Comment on assertive techniques and clarity of presentation. Also encourage discussion of power and its uses.
- Divide into small groups and present each with some advocacy and empowerment case studies, asking group members to analyse the risks in each and identify ways of eliminating or minimising those risks.
- Ask group members to come to the next session prepared to present a case study account of occasions when they have tried to act as advocates on behalf of patients, either successfully or unsuccessfully. Suggest background reading on the debate about independent advocacy versus advocacy by health care professionals.

Day 4

Aims

To review skills in speaking out on behalf of patients and to summarise key areas of risk.

Objectives

At the end of the day each participant will be able to do the following:

(1) Accept and learn from supervision in advocacy
(2) Explain the main legal judgements and statutes affecting patients' rights
(3) Practise skills in speaking out as an advocate
(4) Make plans to eliminate or minimise risks in advocacy
(5) Identify alternative sources of advocacy for patients.

Teaching plan

Morning

- Divide into pairs or threesomes and run a supervision session on the examples of advocacy set as homework from the previous session. Ask supervisors to pay particular attention to advocates' ability to identify risks and make plans to eliminate or minimise them. At the end re-form the large group and discuss not only the learning points arising about advocacy, but also the value and importance of continuing supervision. Check that all group members have access to someone who can act as a supervisor in relation to advocacy issues in the future.
- Tutor or external speaker to present the legal position on patients' rights. Expand into a discussion of additional rights which are not legally enforceable, but which have a strong basis in health charters or in general morality.

Afternoon

- Set up some short scenarios on advocacy, concentrating on the issue of how to speak out assertively on behalf of patients. One way of doing this is for the tutor to describe a situation and read out a comment from a person in power, e.g. a doctor saying, 'I've written the prescription and I'm not prepared to change it now'. Group members then immediately write down what they would say in reply. Go round the group with each person giving a reply. Then ask the group members individually to identify which reply each one preferred. This can be used as the basis for a wider ranging discussion on the nature of assertive behaviour in advocacy situations.
- Tutor to review the resources available for advocates, including alternative agencies which may be able to help in specific situations.

- Group members to evaluate the course, both in terms of personal learning and satisfaction with the teaching methods.

Assessment

The nature and depth of the assessment of trainee advocates will depend on their previous experience and the circumstances in which they will be working, particularly the extent to which they will have ready access to supervision. Many university courses have moved away from an examination system to a modular system with assignments at regular intervals which can also be used to bring performance evidence from practice into the assessment process. Assuming a short module on advocacy worth 10–20 credits towards the second or third year of a first degree, a written assignment of 1500–3000 words is likely to be prescribed. A weakness of non-NVQ programmes is that they tend to rely on academic evidence of competence, rather than direct observation of practice. However, many NVQ programmes have also come to rely less on time-consuming and hard-to-verify observation methods, instead preferring to ask candidates to build up portfolios of written evidence of their competence. A compromise for a taught module is to set an essay, which must be supported by additional written evidence of competence. The marking scheme would depend on the academic level of the module and the preferences of the course team. Stronger weighting could, for example, be attached to risk management or to learning from supervision. A sample essay question using a portfolio is:

> Present a portfolio of evidence of your work as an advocate containing the following:
>
> (1) An example of your work in empowering a patient/client
> (2) An example of your work as an advocate in speaking out on behalf of a different patient/client
> (3) A report, either written or tape recorded, of a supervision session in which advocacy situations are discussed.
>
> Then write a 1500 word analysis of the material in your portfolio, relating it to the advocacy flowchart and bringing out the strengths and weaknesses of your performance as an advocate.

No matter how thoroughly competence is assessed, an introductory advocacy course can only be a first step in developing expertise and safe practice. Continuing review of casework is essential, both as part of periodic continuing education activities and within regular and ongoing supervision.

Summary of key points

- Well-designed initial and continuing education opportunities for advocates are essential
- There are two broad approaches to curriculum design: one relies on detailed specification of competences and the other is based on outline objectives or statements of desired outcomes
- These two approaches may be combined, with the objectives shaping the teaching process and the competences used to strengthen the final assessment by obliging trainees to provide casework evidence of their performance.

Chapter 14
Case Studies

This chapter presents ten case studies to supplement those already quoted in earlier chapters. They are all either written or tape recorded accounts of advocacy given by a variety of advocates. Most were collected in preparation for multidisciplinary training courses over several years and involving staff from several different areas. Some details have been changed to preserve confidentiality and anonymity and they are all used with the permission of the individuals who recounted them. Each example begins with an outline of the background, then the actions of the advocate are described and finally some key points are listed to raise questions for further thought or debate. They could be used or adapted when teaching advocacy, for example by presenting the outline and then asking students what they would do in each situation, before showing them the actions actually taken and discussing the outcomes.

Family problems and the police

A written account provided by a GP.

Outline

'The individual concerned was an Asian man in his sixties whose wife had died some years previously. He had several sons, one of whom was living at home with him, and a teenage daughter who looked after her father devotedly. Before becoming ill with cancer he had worked in a local supermarket but his sons were unemployed. Unfortunately one of the sons was frequently in trouble with the police. As his illness progressed the father needed increasingly frequent periods of respite care in the local hospital, so I would visit him as soon as possible after he came home. It was on one such occasion that I arrived to find him very upset and shaken. Apparently

139

his son was suspected by the police of having committed some mis-demeanour so they had gone in force to the father's house looking for him. Unfortunately the father had only been home from hospital half an hour when the police arrived. He explained the situation as best he could to the police, although this was difficult because they found his accent hard to understand. They went away again but it left him very shaken and dreading something similar might happen at night. We talked the situation over, during which time he said plaintively that "my boys are nothing but trouble to me".'

Actions

'I asked him if he would like me to telephone the senior police officer and explain the situation about his illness, his frequent need to go into hospital and his anxiety. I felt sorry for him and knew he would not be able to do all the explaining needed himself. He said he had no objection to my disclosing that he had cancer. I duly telephoned the police station, told them who I was and said that I wished to speak to a senior officer about one of my patients. The inspector was very understanding. He knew the family well. He said that in future my patient would not be troubled if his son was needed for questioning. He had heard that my patient had been ill and my phone call confirmed the seriousness of his condition, which helped increase the officer's sympathy for him. My patient was greatly relieved when I reported back to him and was not troubled by the police again during his few remaining weeks of life.'

Key points

- This is an example of inter-agency cooperation based on a sympa-thetic understanding of an individual's health condition.
- The doctor volunteered to act as an advocate because he did not believe the patient would be effective in speaking up for himself. Involvement of other family members was ruled out by the nature of the situation.
- The doctor took care to check that the patient would allow him to share his medical details with an outsider.
- The use of power is well illustrated by the way the doctor was able to insist on talking to a senior police officer straight away, by-passing the usual lines of authority.
- The advocacy was successful and involved relatively low risks to the parties involved.

Facial surgery

A written account provided by an enrolled nurse working in a surgical ward.

Outline

'The patient was a 67 year old woman suffering from cancer. She had already had surgery on her tongue and was now facing major facial surgery involving facial disfigurement. Treatment would only be palliative as she had leukaemia and her condition was very unstable. Over the past two years since initial surgery her quality of life had gone down. She had a very supportive son and daughter but was a widow and lived alone. I wondered why in the event of such a poor prognosis this very pleasant lady was undergoing such major trauma for palliative treatment.'

Actions

'I spoke to other members of staff about this case. It seemed to me that such radical surgery could well end her life. The other members of staff felt the same so I approached the consultant. He was pleased that we were so concerned for the wellbeing of our patient. He explained that the surgery was the wish of the patient and the son and daughter agreed with what their mother wanted. The cancer was likely to come through the face in the near future without the surgery. We asked whether she fully understood that she would spend the rest of her life on parenteral feeding and would she be able to cope on her own. The surgeon said he had explained all this to her and she still wanted to go ahead.

The patient had her major surgery. She is still alive and has yet to return to the ward from intensive care. I felt I was successful in presenting my case to the consultant who acccepted all the points I raised. Ultimately I was trying to understand and care for the patient who, although she knew diagnosis and prognosis, chose to ignore the dangers of surgery. I was unsuccessful in preventing the operation as it was the patient's own wish.'

Key points

● Was this advocacy at all? The nurse appeared to be raising her own questions with the consultant without checking with the patient first.

The example can be used to clarify interpretations of what advocacy is about.

- In ethical terms it illustrates the primacy of respect for autonomy over beneficence/non-maleficence in this situation. Because the patient chose the surgery for herself, her wishes had to be respected.
- Would the situation have been the same in reverse – if the patient had seemed reluctant to undergo surgery which the consultant and family recommended? How would the advocacy role of the nurse have changed in those circumstances?

Empowering a mother

A written account provided by a health visitor.

Outline

'I called in to see a mother whose son had speech problems which were affecting his behaviour. It was putting the whole family under a severe strain. I had referred the boy to speech therapy about six months before and he had been seen for assessment, but he was told that he would have to go on a waiting list. I agreed with the mother that the boy needed seeing soon because his speech problems were causing difficulties in relationships across the whole family. The mother wasn't sure what to do and asked me if she should write to her MP.'

Actions

'I said that writing to her MP could do no harm and suggested some of the points she should make in the letter. Some time later a letter addressed to me arrived from the House of Commons. I opened it to find a complaint from the MP that the boy had not received speech therapy and suggesting that I should have got the GP to refer the boy instead of doing it myself (implying that a GP referral would have had more weight).

I was furious and considered writing straight back to the MP, telling him how ignorant I thought he was. However, I took a deep breath and contacted my senior manager, showing her the letter. She suggested it would be better if she took the letter and replied on behalf of the Trust. A calm explanatory letter was sent, stating that the problem was nothing to do with the route of referral. A little while later more speech therapy resources became available and the boy was treated. I do not know if this was the result of the MP's letter or was purely coincidental.'

Key points

- A clear case of empowerment in which the health visitor enabled the mother to make out a case for herself, with eventual success
- It illustrates that there are risks, even in empowerment
- The second stage of seeking advice from a senior manager was a good way of containing the risk to the individual once it had arisen
- Useful for debate about alternative courses of action.

Acting as advocate for a child

A written account provided by a social worker.

Outline

'I was visiting a single mother with a very young baby. The mother had poor parenting skills and a history of sexual abuse by her father. She frequently called us asking for help. On this occasion she said that she was afraid she might harm her baby if things got any worse. I asked her if she had ever done anything to the baby before. She said that she had twice hit him in the ribs with a clenched fist in a fit of temper to stop him crying. But then in tears she said she realised what she had done, cuddled him and comforted him. She said she couldn't bear any harm to come to him.'

Actions

'I told her that I have a legal duty to make a record of what she had said and that there would have to be a case conference to discuss what had happened. But I also told her that I would try to make sure she received the help and support she needed for herself and her son. I think she was shocked that I was taking it further. She said she thought I was her friend and she was telling me these things so I could get her some help, not so that her baby would be taken away from her.

A case conference was held and the health visitor said she had found some marks on the child immediately before the conference and that the mother admitted biting her son. The outcome of the case conference was successful in my opinion in that all the services involved agreed a regular pattern of visits and support with a care plan agreed by everyone including the mother. The child remained with her mother, who felt more secure, although she did ask for the health visitor to be appointed as her key worker rather than me.'

Key points

- The social worker made an assumption about the child's wants and acted as advocate for the child in calling the case conference
- This action appears to have caused some damage to the trust between the social worker and the mother, since she asked for a different key worker
- Advocates need to be clear where their advocacy duty lies in family situations, when they may come under pressure to divide their loyalties. The advocate in this example had no hesitation in seeing the child, and not the mother, as her client.

Patient with a cancer diagnosis

A written account provided by a ward manager.

Outline

'This patient was admitted for investigations and stabilisation of her medical condition. She told me she thought there might be something seriously wrong with her and wanted to know the truth as she had a family to think about. On investigation she was found to have cancer of the colon with bone metastases. Our consultant was reluctant to tell the patient her full diagnosis and prognosis. During the ward round he said she had a "little problem with her bowel".'

Actions

'I spoke to the consultant on his own at the end of the round and said it would be better with this patient to use clearer terms and go back and answer any questions she had about diagnosis or prognosis more directly. I told him she already felt there was a drastic problem with her bowel and she just wanted confirmation. We both went back to her and she asked him if she had cancer. He gave her a true answer and told her that her prognosis was poor although no one could tell her exactly how long she had left. She was very distressed and afraid, but still thanked us for being honest with her. I went back to her later and over the next few days was able to help her plan for the future. I helped her to contact social services to make provision for housing arrangements and also helped her contact a solicitor to write a will to ensure her immediate family were provided for. Despite her distress I feel that I chose the correct course. She has accepted her condition and started to make plans for her limited future.'

Key points

- The example illustrates speaking up for a patient and then empowering her
- The patient had told the nurse what she wanted in advance of the test results, giving her a mandate for advocacy
- The nurse appears to have anticipated some of the risks of confronting the consultant in front of other people; she chose her words carefully when she spoke
- Ethical issues surrounding disclosure can be brought in by asking how the ward manager should have acted if the consultant had argued that the patient was not in a fit condition to accept her full diagnosis and prognosis
- The example can be used to discuss the value of building credibility and expert power by asking what effect the nurse's actions may have had on her relationship with this consultant in the future.

A case conference

A tape recorded account provided by an independent advocate.

Outline

'I can remember one particular time where a case conference had been called at a day unit to talk about a lady aged 75 who had social living conditions that were causing concern to the GP, the social worker and the district nurse. They all thought the lady would be safer if she moved into residential accommodation. Her home was in a poor condition, damp and ramshackle and in an isolated rural area with no public transport. The house was very dirty and untidy. I'd been round to visit as part of our advocacy service for the elderly. I found her perfectly alert and she seemed to manage OK for herself, she just wasn't fussed about hygiene and cleanliness like the rest of us. I put the options to her about going into sheltered accommodation or a residential home but she said, "No thank you". Her husband had been poorly and he had to go into a residential home and I asked if she had considered going to the same place as him but she just said, "Thank you very much, I'm stopping here". So when she came to the day unit there was a case conference and all these other agencies were there discussing what was best. And the lady was sitting beside me. She was hard of hearing and turned to me and said in her broad country dialect, "What are they doing, me duck?".'

Actions

'I said to her, "They're here to talk about your problems". She turned to me and said, "What problems? I ain't got no problems." So I interrupted what was going on in the group and said, "Excuse me. I don't know what you're all here to discuss but this lady hasn't got any problems!" Everybody was there with the best of intentions to discuss this lady's "appalling" living conditions, but she herself was quite happy, thank you very much, and said so herself. She wasn't putting anybody at risk, except perhaps herself. She's still living at home and coming into the day unit about twice a week.'

Key points

- The example brings out the judgement which potential advocates have to make about how far they support the client's wants; the advocate would have chosen differently for herself but accepted the client's right to do what she wanted
- The example can be used for debate about the extent to which professionals allow their own value judgements to influence decisions they take that influence the lives of others
- The example illustrates the value of having an independent advocate who can speak out very directly to professional staff.

A client attending a psychiatric day unit

Two tape-recorded accounts provided by a staff nurse and the patient himself.

Outline

'This particular patient came in looking surly. His face was downcast whereas normally he smiles. It was his general manner that told me something was wrong, but that's only because of having known him for over a year. If he had been a total stranger, it would have been more difficult. So I approached him and it turned out he was particularly dissatisfied with social services. He wanted to do some voluntary work but social services in his area had told him there wasn't any, or at least that's what he said. He had worked in the past, but he had a stroke and that's why he now walked with a slight limp. Plus he had cardiac problems so it was not realistic to point him towards the Job Centre. But he wanted to be of some use to people, instead of being totally useless, so he felt that voluntary work was the best answer. But when he was told that social services couldn't help him, he felt as though that was the end of the story and there was nothing else left for him.'

Actions

'I suggested to him that there are charitable organisations that rely a lot on voluntary workers but don't necessarily want people full time. I also suggested that there are lots of residential homes in the area that might be glad of somebody visiting their residents. And he seemed pleased at this. So I gave him some phone numbers of charities, head offices, and I gave him a copy of Yellow Pages and he began looking at residential homes within easy access for him. And that's all I did. But because he'd got the phone numbers to contact written down, because he'd got that piece of paper, it was something physical for him to hold on to. I wouldn't make the phone calls for him because I didn't want to take away his independence. And in the end he had to meet these people anyway, so I would only have made it harder for him if I did it in the first place. Even a simple phone call to other people, if he can do that, it boosts his ego tremendously. And the next one isn't quite as hard. And that's honestly all I did.'

The client's viewpoint

'And the staff nurse said to me, "Are you alright?" And I said, "I'm bloody not. I'm right sick." But she comes and talks to me and calms me down. She's sorted these telephone numbers out for me, nursing homes and places to see if I can go in and spend a couple of hours with them, helping them voluntary. She got me to write down the telephone numbers so I can ring round and see if I can go there and help them. No money involved. But I could have a game of cards with them or do a bit of washing up. She suggested it, the nurse. I was feeling lousy but then she came down talking to me and it just floats away. You see, I'm having a good day today.'

Key points

- A clear example of empowerment with an explanation of the reason for choosing this course of action rather than telephoning on the patient's behalf
- The nurse played down the value of her actions whereas they were important to the patient
- This was part of a longer term plan for helping the patient to be more independent. It could be used as part of a debate over whether there is a difference between short term advocacy, as is typical in many hospital situations, and the longer term relationships that are possible in community care and independent advocacy.

Helping a patient claim benefit

A tape-recorded account provided by a district nurse.

Outline

'Mr C is 78 years old. He is partially sighted and is in poor health but still lives in his own home. Up until last year he was sexton at the local church, which supplemented his income in a small way and which he very much enjoyed. Failing health and poor eyesight have forced him to relinquish the post, but he now has extra expenses that he can ill afford. He told me that his finances are his main worry at the moment.'

Actions

'I explained that he did have the option of moving to residential care but he was adamant that he wanted to stay in his own home for as long as he can. I felt that he would be eligible for attendance allowance which would help him pay for extra care and visits to a local day centre. He is a proud man and was very reluctant to claim anything. I asked him about his jobs in the past and whether he had paid income tax regularly, which he had. It took a bit of persuading but in the end he agreed that filling in the form only meant claiming what he might be entitled to because of all his years of contributions. We filled in the claim forms together and we are awaiting the result. I am optimistic that he will qualify. I really think he would be better in a residential home but feel I must respect his right to choose for himself.'

Key points

- This is an example of empowering a patient by giving him information and helping him to fill in a claim form
- The nurse mentions 'persuading' and this passage can be used to discuss the extent to which it is legitimate for an advocate to urge a particular course of action on a client
- The example also provides another illustration of the importance of respect for autonomy in all forms of advocacy.

An operation under local anaesthetic

A written account provided by a staff nurse on a surgical ward.

Outline

'While admitting a patient for a total hip replacement it became obvious that she was very anxious. It turned out that the main reason for her anxiety was the fact that 20 years ago both her sisters had died after undergoing surgery and both had had spinal anaesthetics. She was thinking that the same would happen to her if she had a spinal anaesthetic.'

Actions

'After she had explained her fears I held her hand, which seemed to give her a little reassurance. I told her I would personally speak to the anaesthetist and tell him about her fears. I also explained that things have changed dramatically over the past 20 years and that anaesthetics are much safer now. At the end of our talk she seemed calmer.

The anaesthetist came the following day half an hour before the lady was due to go to theatre. I told him about her anxieties about a spinal anaesthetic but he took it upon himself to tell her that was what he intended to do. She was not given a pre-med and ended up crying and very upset. The anaesthetist totally ignored my reasoning and I felt that in some way I had let the patient down. No way could I persuade her that it was best to have a spinal anaesthetic.'

Key points

- An obvious starting point is whether the nurse had really let the patient down. The fact that this example does not really give enough information to make a full judgement possible can be used to ask what information would be needed. For example, was there anything in the woman's medical history that made a general anaesthetic risky? Did the nurse consider speaking to the anaesthetist earlier so that these decisions were not being made at the last minute? Was empowerment considered fully, for example at the time the consent form was signed?

- The example also demonstrates the difficulty of a professional acting as an advocate within an employing organisation. On the other hand, is independent advocacy really feasible on busy surgical wards?

Protest for the inner child

A written account by a community psychiatric nurse.

Outline

'I was working with a woman over about a year. She had been abused as a child, not physical or sexual abuse but being "used" by her parents as a pawn in their relationship games. The father was a dominant and rather aggressive man. The mother was more submissive but was also rather manipulative. The mother sought to avoid sexual intercourse with the father by making her daughter dependent on her. She encouraged her daughter to say she was afraid of being alone in the dark and to ask to sleep in the same bed with her parents. In my opinion the mother was using her daughter both literally and metaphorically as a barrier between her and her husband. The woman grew up anxious and submissive. She became anxious whenever she was faced with even minor problems in her life and sought help from her GP who referred her to me.'

Actions

'As I worked with her I tried to help her to see for herself what had happened to her. At the end of nine months she had achieved an intellectual understanding of this, recognising that she had been used in parental power games. She still visited her parents regularly and worried about the visits. I gently tried to help her to find small things that she could take a stand on to help her to develop a feeling of independence, but once there she never could say what she planned. I feel that I was trying to be an advocate for the inner child inside of her, to help her to recognise what had happened to that inner child and then for her to speak out for herself.

She was already very submissive and I decided it would only do harm if I tried to push her to stand up for herself any more than I had done, so I was feeling disappointed in the end with no real changes being achieved that I could see. But the woman had a child of her own who was about four years old. One day they were visiting the parents, who were having a big argument. The woman's mother started telling her father to be quiet because he was disturbing her grandchild who was very delicate and could not stand a lot of noise and disruption. Suddenly the daughter could see the old power game being played out again right before her eyes, but this time with her own daughter as the pawn. She became absolutely furious at what her parents were doing. She jumped up and vented her rage on both of them. Then she took her child away and had no contact with the parents for several months. For her it had been a turning point. Although she had never been able to stand up for her own inner child, she was able to protest as an advocate for her biological child. In a sense I think she was protesting for herself as well.'

Key points

- This is a powerful example of empowerment leading to advocacy on behalf of self and another
- It illustrates a counselling approach which forms part of many empowering interventions
- The meaning of advocacy for the inner child may give rise to a useful discussion
- The example also offers hope that people really can learn and change through empowering advocacy.

Chapter 15
The Way Forward

It is a pity that advocacy continues to be so necessary in health care; it is a pity that the rights of patients and clients are still not always accepted by the professionals, some of whom prefer to equate illness with a state of childlike dependence; it is also a pity that the legal position in the UK still supports a paternalistic interpretation of the role of doctors in relation both to patients and to other professionals. Moreover there is a cultural problem built into medical education which takes the genuine human concern of student doctors and all too frequently distorts it into a more remote, scientific attitude to the human body and human behaviour. Beyond this, there is a political problem built into the way the National Health Service is organised, which allows unrepresentative and unelected groups the freedom to 'commission' health services on behalf of the population of a local area which has no real power to exercise any positive influence over decisions. Finally, it is a pity that patients continue on the whole to be very willing to place naive trust in the professionals and very reluctant to demand more information about their own treatment and care.

If the above assertions are accepted, they represent a situation which professionals, politicians and patients can (and in my view should) campaign to change for the better. But in the meantime patients – and we are all potential patients – need people inside and outside the service who are prepared to offer advocacy on their behalf, as a counter-balance to those in authority and to the system which confers that authority. The trouble is that wherever advocacy is most needed, it is also most risky. The patients are at risk from bungled advocacy and from advocacy with a hidden agenda which is not their own; the professionals in authority are at risk from unduly confrontational advocacy which leaves a trail of bitter feelings and damaged reputations in its wake; and the advocates themselves are at risk from a system which all too easily equates advocacy with disloyalty and trouble making.

Fortunately it is possible to limit these risks, making advocacy safer and more effective for all concerned. Promotion of self-advocacy comes top of the list. To the extent that patients and clients can be empowered to speak up for themselves there is a double benefit. First they have ultimate authority over their own minds and bodies, with strong rights to say 'no' or 'not yet', and so can force the professionals to stop and listen to what they want in situations where the claims of external advocates would not be heard. Secondly, and as part of the process, the patients learn how to exercise and extend their rights while at the same time conditioning the professionals to accept the corresponding duty of respect for autonomy.

After self-advocacy comes independent advocacy. People from outside the health care system bring a fresh perspective and respond differently because they are not part of the hierarchical culture of the complex organisations in which modern health care is delivered. Provided their funding is safe from undue interference from within the health care system, independent advocates are relatively invulnerable in their work, because the professionals cannot easily use position or resource power against them. This is the main reason why access to independent advocacy is a necessary part of a comprehensive health care service. It is not that the advocates are any better at working with clients than the professionals, nor do they have better training or supervision. Indeed there is just as much scope for abuse, hidden agendas and ineffective working within independent advocacy as there is when professionals take on the role. The difference is the lower level of risk to the independent advocate, which allows a greater freedom of speech and action, with significant benefits for clients and all concerned.

Independent advocacy has always emphasised the establishment of longer-term partnerships with vulnerable clients. Yet many people need short-term or crisis advocacy when their health becomes impaired. This is where advocacy by professionals comes into its own. It is undoubtedly the most risky form of advocacy, but in my opinion it will always be a necessary part of the role of all health care professionals. Their large numbers, expert knowledge and ability to network mean that professionals who are willing to act as advocates are a vital support to patients and clients in all specialties and in both hospital and community settings. However, many of the examples cited in this book have clearly established the limitations and drawbacks to safe working by professionals. What I hope is that some of the examples have also shown a way forward.

Risk management in this area means having a clear view of the realities of power in any given situation and then consciously trading on this knowledge. The establishment of expert power is particularly important and can also be allied to personal power to the extent that individuals consider it ethical to use it. Anticipation of risk is vital. It is not enough to rush into situations with the crusading zeal of someone who can see an injustice and is determined to put it right. Effective advocacy demands a clear head as well as a strong heart. The risks need to be identified and then actions taken to minimise or eliminate them. All helpers must come to recognise that in an advocacy career there are bound to be times when the risks are just too great and external advocacy is simply not possible. It is surely better to conserve one's strength for another day than to sacrifice all one's future clients in a futile gesture that only results in conflict for its own sake. However, ultimately each of us must make our own decisions. Advocacy is certainly about power, but it is also about a concern for fairness and a close emotional identification with people who are vulnerable. Seen in these terms advocacy ceases to be something separate from everyday experience; instead it becomes an integral part of the caring enterprise which is a health service.

References

Albarran, J.W. (1992) Advocacy in critical care – an evaluation of the implications for nurses and the future. *Intensive Critical Care Nursing*, **8** (1), 47–53.

Allen I., Hogg D. & Peace S. (1992) *Elderly People: Choice, Participation and Satisfaction*. Policy Studies Institute, London.

Allmark, P. & Klarzynski, R. (1992) The case against nurse advocacy. *British Journal of Nursing*, **2** (1), 33–6.

Balint, M. (1964) *The Doctor, His Patient and the Illness*. Pitman Medical Limited, London.

Beardshaw, V. (1981) Complaints about ill treatment. In *Conscientious Objectors at Work* (ed. V. Beardshaw). Social Audit, London.

Beauchamp, T.L. & Childress, J.F. (1979) *Principles of Biomedical Ethics*. Oxford University Press, New York.

Becker, P. (1986) Advocacy in nursing: perils and possibilities. *Holistic Nursing Practice*, **1** (1), 54–63.

Booth, W. (1991) A cry for help in the wilderness. *Health Service Journal*, **101** (5238), 26–7.

Brower, H.T. (1982) Advocacy: what it is. *Journal of Gerontological Nursing*, **8** (3), 141–3.

Brown, J. & Ritchie, J.A. (1990) Nurses' perceptions of parents' and nurses' roles in caring for hospitalised children. *Children's Health Care*, **19** (1), 28–36.

Cabell, C. (1992) The efficacy of primary nursing as a foundation for patient advocacy. *Nursing Practice*, **5** (3), 2–5.

Cahill, J. (1994) Are you prepared to be their advocate? *Professional Nurse*, **9** (6), 371–5.

Callery, P. (1995) *An investigation into the role of parents in the care of hospitalised children*. PhD thesis, Liverpool University.

Care Sector Consortium (1992) *Mental Health Care: Care Awards Level 3*. Ref no SS0085, Local Government Management Board, London.

Carpenter, D. (1992) Advocacy. *Nursing Times*, **88** (27), i–viii.

Castledine, G. (1981) The nurse as patient's advocate: pros and cons. *Nursing Mirror*, **153** (20), 38–40.

Chaudhary, V. (1991) Avoidable injuries, infrequent washes ... a catalogue of shame and neglect. *The Guardian*, 9 July.

157

Clarke, M. (1989) Guest editorial: patient/client advocacy. *Journal of Advanced Nursing*, **14**, 513–14.

Corcoran, S. (1986) Decision analysis: a step-by-step guide for making clinical decisions. *Nursing Health Care*, **7**, 149–54.

Corcoran, S. (1994) Toward operationalizing an advocacy role. In *Contemporary Leadership Behavior: Selected Readings* (eds E.C. Hein & M.J. Nicholson), 4th edn. pp.153–62. J.B. Lippincott Company, Philadelphia.

Cornwell, J. & Gordon, P. (eds) (1984) *An experiment in advocacy: the Hackney multi-ethnic women's health project*. Report of a conference held on 4 June 1984 at The King's Fund Centre, London.

Copp, L.A. (1986), The nurse as advocate for vulnerable persons. *Journal of Advanced Nursing*, **11** (3), 255–63.

Coyne, I.T. (1995) Parental participation in care: a critical review of the literature. *Journal of Advanced Nursing*, **21** (4), 716–22.

Cresswell, J. & Davies, P. (1992) Give a little whistle? *Health Service Journal*, **102** (5315), 14.

Cross, M. (1994) Draft NHS code of confidentiality 'lacks substance', say objectors. *Health Service Journal*, **104** (5416), 5.

Curtin, L.L. (1979) The nurse as advocate: a philosophical foundation for nursing. *Advances in Nursing Science*, **3**, 1–10.

Dawson, P. & Palmer, W. (1991) *Self-Advocacy at Work*. EMFEC (originally East Midlands Further Education Council), Nottingham.

Darbyshire, P. (1992) *Parenting in public: a study of the experience of parents who live-in with their hospitalised child, and of their relationships with paediatric nurses*. PhD thesis, University of Edinburgh.

Department of Health (1992) *The Patient's Charter*. HMSO, London.

Dexter, G. & Russell, J. (1995) Client centred supervision. In *Psychiatric Nursing Skills* (eds G. Dexter & M. Wash). Chapman Hall, London.

Dickson, A. (1982) *A Woman in Your Own Right*. Quartet Books, London.

Dimond, B. (1993) *Accountability, the Law and the Nurse*. Distance Learning Centre, South Bank University, London.

Dingwall, R. (1983) Introduction. In *The Sociology of the Professions* (eds R. Dingwall & P. Lewis). Macmillan, London.

Drummond, H. (1990) *Managing Difficult People*. Kogan Page, London.

Elliott Pennels, C.J. (1998) Consent and adults. *Professional Nurse*, **13** (4), 252–3.

Fay, P. (1978) Sounding board – in support of patient advocacy as a nursing role. *Nursing Outlook*, **26** (4), 252–3.

Gadow, S. (1980a) Existential advocacy: philosophical foundation of nursing. In *Nursing: Images and Ideals* (eds S.F. Spicker & S. Gadow). Springer, New York.

Gadow, S. (1980b) A model for ethical decision making. *Oncology Nursing Forum*, **7** (3), 44–7.

Gates, B. (1994) *Advocacy: A Nurses' Guide*. Scutari, London.

Gates, B. (1995) Whose best interest? *Nursing Times*, **91** (4), 31–2.

Gibson, C.H. (1995) The process of empowerment in mothers of chronically ill children. *Journal of Advanced Nursing*, **21** (6), 1201–10.

Graham, A. (1992) Advocacy: what the future holds. *British Journal of Nursing*, **1** (3), 148–58.

Handy, C. (1985) *Understanding Organizations*. Penguin, Harmondsworth.

Hayward, J. (1975) *Information – A Prescription Against Pain*. Royal College of Nursing, London.

Health Service Journal (1993) Chapman returns to NHS work. *Health Service Journal*, **103** (5374), 6.

Herzlich, C. (1973) *Health and Illness*. Academic Press, New York.

Hugill, B. (1992), Fraud probe after hospital sacks its whistle-blower. *The Observer*, 11 October.

Hunt, G. & Shailer, B. (1995) Chapter 1 in *Whistleblowing in the Health Service* (ed. G. Hunt). Edward Arnold, London.

Jenny, J. (1979) Patient advocacy – another role for nursing? *International Nursing Review*, **26** (6), 176–81.

Jones, E.W. (1982) Advocacy – a tool for radical nursing curriculum planners. *Journal of Nurse Education*, **21** (1), 40–45.

Kendrick, K. (1994) An advocate for whom – doctor or patient? *Professional Nurse*, **9** (12), 826–9.

Kohnke, M.F. (1982) *Advocacy: Risk and Reality*. The CV Mosby Company, St Louis.

Kolb, D. (1984) *Experiential Learning*. Prentice Hall, New Jersey.

Love, C (1996a) Using a diary to learn the patient's perspective. *Professional Nurse*, **11** (5), 286–8.

Malin, N. & Teasdale, K. (1991) Caring versus empowerment: considerations for nursing practice. *Journal of Advanced Nursing*, **16**, 657–62.

Mallik, M.A. (1995) *Advocacy in nursing*. MPhil thesis, Nottingham University.

Mallik, M. (1997) Advocacy in nursing – perceptions of practising nurses. *Journal of Clinical Nursing*, **6** (4), 303–13.

Mallik, M. & McHale, J. (1995) Support for advocacy. *Nursing Times*, **91** (4), 31–2.

McFadyen, J.A. (1989) Who will speak out for me? *Nursing Times*, **85** (6), 45–8.

Melia, K. (1989) *Everyday Nursing Ethics*. Macmillan, London.

Mihill, C. (1991) Nurse in staffing row faces sack. *The Guardian*, 9 July.

Miles, A. (1984) The stigma of psychiatric disorder. In *Psychiatric Services in the Community* (eds J. Reed & G Lomas). Croom Helm, London.

Miller, B.K., Mansen, T.J. & Lee, H. (1983) Patient advocacy: do nurses have the power and authority to act as patient advocate? *Nursing Leadership*, **6** (2), 56–60.

Miller, S. (1979) Controllability and human stress: method, evidence and theory. *Behaviour Research and Therapy*, **17** (4), 287–304.

Miller, S., Combs, C. & Stoddard, E. (1989) Information, coping and control in patients undergoing surgery and stressful medical procedures. In *Stress, Personal Control and Health* (eds A. Steptoe & A. Appels), pp. 107–30. John Wiley & Sons Ltd, Chichester.

Morrison, A. (1991) The nurse's role in relation to advocacy. *Nursing Standard*, **5** (41), 37–40.

Morse, J.M. (1991) Negotiating commitment and involvement in the nurse–patient relationship. *Journal of Advanced Nursing,* **16** (4), 455–68.

NCVQ (1997) *The Awarding Bodies' Common Accord.* National Council for Vocational Qualifications, London.

Nelson, M. (1988) Advocacy in nursing. *Nursing Outlook,* **36** (3), 136–41.

Nelson-Jones, R. (1989) *Practical Counselling and Helping Skills.* Cassell, London.

Parsons, L. & Day, S. (1992) Improving obstetric outcomes in ethnic minorities: an evaluation of health advocacy in Hackney. *Journal of Public Health Medicine,* **14** (2), 183–91.

Parsons, T. (1951) Illness and the role of the physician: a sociological analysis. *American Journal of Orthopsychiatry,* **21**, 452–60.

Porter, S. (1988) Siding with the system. *Nursing Times,* **84** (41), 30–31.

Proctor, B. (1991) On being a trainer. In *Training and Supervision for Counselling in Action* (eds W. Dryden & B. Thorne), pp. 49–73. Sage, London.

Public Concern at Work (1997) *A Review of the Activities of Public Concern at Work.* 16 Baldwin Gardens, London.

Robinson, D. (1972) Illness, behaviour and children's hospitalisation: a schema of parents' attitudes towards authority. *Social Science and Medicine,* **6**, 447–68.

Robinson, M.B. (1985) Patient advocacy and the nurse: is there a conflict of interest? *Nursing Forum,* **22** (2), 58–63.

Rogers, C.R. (1957) The necessary and sufficient conditions of psycho-therapeutic personality change. *Journal of Consulting Psychology,* **21**, 95–103.

Sang, B. & O'Brien, J. (1984) *Advocacy: the UK and American Experiences.* Project Paper No. 51, The King's Fund Centre, London.

Schon, D.A. (1983) *The Reflective Practitioner. How Professionals Think in Action.* Temple Smith, London.

Segesten, K. (1993) Patient advocacy – an important part of the daily work of the expert nurse. *Scholarly Inquiry for Nursing Practice,* **7** (2), 129–35.

Simons, K. (1992) Who counts? *Community Care: Inside Supplement,* **908**, 26 March, iv–v.

Southgate, J. (1988) The practice of the therapist advocate. *Journal of the Institute for Self-Analysis,* **2** (1), 21–9.

Stockwell, F. (1984) *The Unpopular Patient.* Croom Helm, London.

Sutor, J. (1993) Can nurses be effective advocates? *Nursing Standard,* **7** (22), 30–32.

Teasdale, K. (ed) (1991) *Notes on Advocacy.* Pilgrim Hospital, Boston, Lincolnshire.

Teasdale, K. (ed) (1992a) *Managing the Changes in Health Care.* Wolfe, London.

Teasdale, K. (1992b) *Reassurance in nursing.* PhD thesis, Sheffield Hallam University.

Teasdale, K. (1994) Advocacy and the nurse manager. *Journal of Nursing Management,* **2**, 93–7.

Teasdale, K. (1995) Theoretical and practical considerations on the use of reassurance in the nursing management of anxious patients. *Journal of Advanced Nursing*, **22**, 79–86.

Teasdale, K. & Teasdale, S. (1996) Nursing on the Internet. *Professional Nurse*, **12** (3), 181–4.

Thorne, S.E. & Robinson, C.A. (1988) Reciprocal trust in health care relationships. *Journal of Advanced Nursing*, **13**, 782–9.

Thorold, O. (1981) Nurse whistleblowers and the law. In *Conscientious Objectors at Work* (ed. V. Beardshaw). Social Audit, London.

UKCC (1989) *Exercising Accountability.* United Kingdom Central Council for Nursing, Midwifery and Health Visiting, London.

UKCC (1992) *Code of Professional Conduct*, 3rd edn. United Kingdom Central Council for Nursing, Midwifery and Health Visiting, London.

Waterson, J. (1993) Keeping Mum. *Health Service Journal*, **103** (533), 27–9.

Webb, C. (1987) Professionalism revisited. *NursingTimes*, **83**, 39–41.

Wertheimer, A (1993) *Speaking Out: Citizen Advocacy and Older People.* Centre for Policy on Ageing, London.

White, K. (1990) The little caretaker self. *Journal of the Institute for Self-Analysis*, **4** (1), 38–41.

Whittaker, A. (1988) A voice of their own. *KF News: The Newsletter of the King's Fund*, **11**, 4.

Whittaker, A. (1990) Involving people with learning difficulties in meetings. In *Power to the People: the Key to Responsive Services in Health and Social Care* (ed. King's Fund Centre), pp. 41–8. King's Fund, London.

Wilson Barnett, J. & Carrigy, A. (1978) Factors influencing patients' emotional responses to hospitalisation. *Journal of Advanced Nursing*, **3**, 221–9.

Winslow, G.R. (1984) From loyalty to advocacy: a new metaphor for nursing. *The Hastings Centre Report*, June, 32–40.

Wolfensberger, W. (1972) The Principles of Normalization in Human Services. National Institute on Mental Retardation, Toronto.

Wynne-Harley, D., Teasdale, K., Evans, G. & Ellis, P. (1996) Can a nurse be a patient's advocate? *Professional Nurse*, **11** (10), 655–8.

Index